Urban transformations and public health in the emergent city

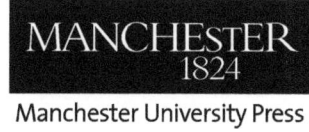

global urban transformations

Series Editors
Michael Keith and Susan Parnell

Urban transformations and public health in the emergent city

Edited by Michael Keith and Andreza Aruska de Souza Santos

Manchester University Press

Copyright © Manchester University Press 2020

While copyright in the volume as a whole is vested in Manchester University Press, copyright in individual chapters belongs to their respective authors.

An electronic version of this book is also available under a Creative Commons (CC-BY-NC-ND) licence, which permits non-commercial use, distribution and reproduction provided the editors, chapter authors and Manchester University Press are fully cited and no modifications or adaptations are made. Details of the licence can be viewed at https://creativecommons.org/licenses/by-nc-nd/4.0/

Published by Manchester University Press
Altrincham Street, Manchester M1 7JA
www.manchesteruniversitypress.co.uk

British Library Cataloguing-in-Publication Data
A catalogue record for this book is available from the British Library

ISBN 978 1 5261 5095 0 hardback
ISBN 978 1 5261 5094 3 open access

First published 2020

The publisher has no responsibility for the persistence or accuracy of URLs for any external or third-party internet websites referred to in this book, and does not guarantee that any content on such websites is, or will remain, accurate or appropriate.

Typeset by
Servis Filmsetting Ltd, Stockport, Cheshire

We would like to dedicate this volume from Andreza to my grandfather, who built Brasilia and taught me to look at cities and see hope; and from Michael to Max and Alex for whom future cities matter.

Contents

Series editors' foreword ix
List of contributors x

1 Introduction: urban transformation and public health in future cities – Michael Keith and Andreza Aruska de Souza Santos 1

2 Mental health, stress and the contemporary metropolis – Nikolas Rose 35

3 Feminised urban futures, healthy cities and violence against women and girls: transnational reflections from Brazilians in London and Maré, Rio de Janeiro – Cathy McIlwaine, Miriam Krenzinger, Yara Evans and Eliana Sousa Silva 55

4 Understanding the relationships between wellbeing and mobility in the unequal city: the case of community initiatives promoting cycling and walking in São Paulo and London – Tim Schwanen and Denver V. Nixon 79

5 Urban (sanitation) transformation in China: a Toilet Revolution and its socio-eco-technical entanglements – Deljana Iossifova 102

6 The food environment and health in African cities: analysing the linkages and exploring possibilities for improving health and wellbeing – Warren Smit 123

7 Urban mental health and the moral economies of suffering in a 'broken city': reinventing depression among Rio de

Janeiro urban dwellers – Leandro David Wenceslau and
   Francisco Ortega 147
8 Violence as a language of construction and deconstruction
   in Rio de Janeiro and Brazil – Luiz Eduardo Soares 171
9 Conclusion: city DNA, public health and a new urban
   imaginary – Michael Keith and Andreza Aruska de Souza
   Santos 198

Index 212

Series editors' foreword

This book series addresses the causes, dynamics and understandings of global urban transformation in the twenty-first century. We live in an era when numerically the greatest number of people moving to cities are in the parts of the globe normally characterised as the global south. It is also the case that in recent years much of the most interesting, innovative and insightful work around contemporary urbanisms has addressed the global condition through a disposition that speaks internationally both from and to this new cartography.

We have put together this series with Manchester University Press to reflect and capture these trends and realities and look for new voices that might articulate and curate these new realities through fresh lenses.

We look to publish work that is:

International, working within a global frame of reference, where cases are generative of larger transnational processes. The series aims to move urban studies to a focus that transcends a traditional separation of literatures of the global south and global north.

Interdisciplinary, originating mostly but not entirely from within the social sciences. The orientation of the series seeks work that rethinks interdisciplinarity in an urban context, drawing on insights from natural sciences and humanities as well as the social sciences.

Informed by the past but future oriented, addressing the challenges of the emergent cities of the twenty-first century. This perspective values the particularities of history and geography; the path dependencies of urban change; and the realities of spatial variation. It recognises the predictive value of new methods of data collection and technological change but considers that such a 'future' city orientation moves beyond extrapolation from trend to a more multidimensional sensibility.

Addressing multiple audiences, working across conventionally defined urban scholarly and professional interests (such as architecture, planning, city politics and urban regeneration), privileging work that has value for city thought leaders and activists, the general reader as well as students and the specialist academic audience.

Multi-scalar, recognising the value of different scales of analysis, commissioning work that focuses on geographies that range from trends in rapidly expanding megacity regions, smaller towns or the dynamics of neighbourhood change.

Multi-actor, welcoming contributions that detail stakeholder interactions that drive urban change, including tracking the power dynamics and institutional politics between residents, civil society, the state, business or traditional authorities.

Michael Keith and Susan Parnell

List of contributors

Andreza Aruska de Souza Santos (Editor) is Director of the Brazilian Studies Programme and Lecturer at the Latin American Centre, University of Oxford. Her work focuses on urban and political anthropology, looking mainly at political participation in contexts of informal economies in small and medium-sized cities. She is the author of the book *Politics of memory: Urban cultural heritage in Brazil* (Rowman & Littlefield, 2019), which examines the relationship between nationalism, collective memory and the making and unmaking of historic cities in Brazil.

Yara Evans is a visiting research associate at King's College London. Her research interests focus on the social and economy dynamics of immigrant communities in the UK, especially the Brazilians, although her recent focus has been on violence against women. She has also a keen interest on animal and human interactions, and enjoys looking after feline and vulpine creatures at her home in London.

Deljana Iossifova is Senior Lecturer in Urban Studies at the University of Manchester. Her research is concerned with questions of urban inequality, coexistence and transformation in China and other transitioning contexts. Most recently, she has investigated uneven urban development through the lens of urban infrasystems, particularly sanitation.

Michael Keith (Editor) is the Director of the PEAK Urban programme on global urban futures, working between China, Colombia, India and South Africa and the Centre on Migration Policy and Society at the

University of Oxford. He was also the Director of the Economic and Social Research Council (ESRC) Urban Transformations Programme (2015–20). His own research has focused on the interface of migration and urbanism. He has experience outside the academy in the fields of city politics and urban regeneration, having held office as the leader of a London local authority and founded and sat on boards of a range of public–private partnerships and urban regeneration companies. He has also spent several decades working with voluntary-sector organisations in inner-city settings, being particularly focused on issues of racial injustice.

Miriam Krenzinger is Director of the School of Social Services at the Federal University of Rio de Janeiro. She has a PhD in social work from the Catholic University of Rio Grande do Sul (PUCRS), where her thesis focused on the need for a more complex examination of the interplay between violence and prisons in contemporary society. She is the author of many books, and her research specialisms also include social work provision and rights for street homeless populations and violence against women and girls.

Cathy McIlwaine is Professor of Development Geography in the Department of Geography, King's College London. Her research focuses on gender and development issues in the global south, and on transnational migration in London with a specific focus on the Latin American community from the perspective of livelihoods, citizenship and gender-based violence. She is also a trustee of the charities Latin Elephant and the Latin American Bureau, and an adviser for the Latin American Women's Rights Service.

Denver V. Nixon is currently an honorary research associate of the Transport Studies Unit at the University of Oxford and teaches in the Department of Geography at the University of British Columbia. His work at Oxford investigates grassroots walking and cycling infrastructural initiatives for marginalized communities in London and São Paulo. More broadly, Nixon is interested in how environmentally (un)sustainable and socially (un)just practices are formed and maintained through embodied experiences and structural contexts.

Francisco Ortega is Full Professor in the Institute for Social Medicine of the State University of Rio de Janeiro and Research Director of the Rio

Center for Global Health. He is also Visiting Professor at the Department of Global Health and Social Medicine of King's College London.

Nikolas Rose is Professor of Sociology in the Department of Global Health and Social Medicine at King's College London and Co-Director of King's ESRC Centre for Society and Mental Health, the UK's first major research centre on the social dimensions of mental distress. His current research concerns the role of the life sciences, neurosciences and psychiatry in changing regimes for governing human beings. His most recent book is *Our psychiatric future: The politics of mental health* (Polity Press, 2018); the next, *The urban brain: Mental health in the vital city*, written with Des Fitzgerald, will be published by Princeton University Press in 2020.

Tim Schwanen is Professor of Transport Studies and Geography and Director of the Transport Studies Unit at the University of Oxford. He is also Fellow in Geography at St Anne's College, Oxford. His research uses the everyday mobilities of people, goods and information as a lens on broader questions about transitions to low-carbon living, climate change, social inequality, health and wellbeing, and scientific knowledge production.

Eliana Sousa Silva, an academic and social activist, has a PhD in social service from PUC-Rio (the Pontifical Catholic University of Rio de Janeiro) and is the Director of the NGO Redes da Maré (Maré Development Networks) in Rio de Janeiro. She is the Curator and Director of the Women of the World Festival in Rio de Janeiro and an advisory board member of the Women of the World Global Foundation. She is also a visiting professor holding the Olavo Setubal Chair in Arts, Culture and Science at the Institute of Advanced Studies of the University of São Paulo and the leader of the CNPq (National Council for Scientific and Technological Development) Research Group Policies Center for Violence Prevention, Access to Justice and Education in Human Rights.

Warren Smit is the manager of research at the African Centre for Cities, University of Cape Town, South Africa. He has a PhD in urban planning and has been a researcher on urban issues for over twenty-five years. His main areas of research include urban health, urban governance and housing policy, with a particular focus on African cities.

Luiz Eduardo Soares is an anthropologist, writer, political scientist, playwright and retired professor at the State University of Rio de Janeiro. He has been a visiting scholar at Harvard University, Columbia University, the University of Virginia and the University of Pittsburgh. He has published seventeen books, among them *Rio de Janeiro: Extreme city* (Penguin, 2016). He has been the Brazilian National Secretary of Public Security, Coordinator of Security, Justice and Citizenship of the State of Rio de Janeiro, and Municipal Secretary of Violence Prevention in Porto Alegre and Nova Iguaçu.

Leandro David Wenceslau is Assistant Professor of Family Medicine in the Department of Nursing and Medicine of the Federal University of Viçosa, Brazil. He is currently a member of the Mental Health Working Group of the Brazilian Society of Family Medicine and of the World Organization of Family Doctors.

1

Introduction: urban transformation and public health in future cities

Michael Keith and Andreza Aruska de Souza Santos

The air we breathe, the climate we share with others and the streets we walk down in the city where we might work and live are all just some of the many forms of *urban commons*. Like all commons they foreground the tensions between social demands that are shared by large numbers and particular rights that might be exercised by individuals, minorities and majorities. Conceptually, the notion of the city commons spans scholarly traditions. They range from empirically oriented political science to strands of critical urban studies informed by Deleuzian and autonomist philosophical and political traditions (compare Berge, Cole and Ostrom, 2012; Hardt and Negri, 2009: 252–6; Amin and Thrift, 2017). How we make sense of what *I might* do and what *we should* do has always been at the heart of the urban condition. But how we sustain the long-term future of economy, ecology and social life in a city that is shared by contemporary demographics and future generations defines the instrumental imperatives of a twenty-first-century planet shaped by urban growth. And for the interests of this volume they particularly shape the chances of living a life that is healthy in the cities of the contemporary moment and the immediate future.[1] The city is both a frame and a container of determinants of public health. The conditioning context of natural and built environments, collective access to food, water and air and diverse regimes of socio-economics and governance define the material framing and *distal* determinants of public health, while it is in the spaces of the urban that the aggregations of individual behaviours, genetic and epigenetic configurations, nutrition and living mediate more *proximal* determinants of longevity and morbidity. Both are addressed by public health systems that in the main try to optimise the wellbeing of the maximum number of individuals in the name of a public good. So as cities increasingly define the human condition, how this public good is realised (or not) through different city forms becomes an issue of expanding scientific enquiry and urgent policy formation.

The dilemmas of city commons form a sub-set of what is known in economics, politics and social policy as 'common pool resource problems' (Olson, 1965), a generic challenge to the normative settlement of urban life. Common pool resource problems address what Hardin (1968) classically identified pessimistically as the 'tragedy of the commons', invoking the possibility of humanity's potential to exhaust and destroy sensitive ecosystems. They also exemplify what the Nobel Prize winner Elinor Ostrom more optimistically identified as the sorts of problems confronted, managed and overcome by humanity in many different moments in time and place across the globe. Ostrom amassed an abundance of empirical exemplifications of common pool resource situations and systems to inform her optimism (Ostrom et al., 2002). And for some, because of the density of multiple forms of use and plural public interests, cities are spaces saturated with people, conflicting uses and private investment that define the urban as a constitutively generic form of commons that can be successfully managed only under appropriate institutional forms of law and governance (Huron, 2015: 977; Foster and Iaione, 2016).

But we also know that city systems are not singular or simple: they are complex and open, social and ecological, systems of systems where urban metabolism, economic dynamics, transport networks and demographic change all reshape one another recursively. And as several scholars have pointed out, there is a literature that tries to combine complex systems theory and common pool resource solutions to the tragedy of the commons, but it is not a literature that is either particularly well developed or invariably optimistic. Indeed it has been argued that common pool resource problems and complex systems thinking have too often been considered apart from one another (Wilson, 2012) and are even more rarely reconciled when the most appropriate structures of governance are considered (Berkes, 2017; Colding and Barthel, 2019). Moreover, it is the combinations of medical aetiologies, normative systems of resource allocation, political systems of governance and social systems of behaviour that structure the living city. Both existing patterns and future determinants of public health thus demand a conversation between social sciences and medical and natural sciences. That conversation is the central concern of this volume.

In this volume we have drawn together a series of contributions that address pressing issues of urban public health. Our starting points are twofold. The first is the recognition that in the twenty-first century the majority of the globe's urban populations will live in cities. The cities of continents that are at the heart of this volume in Latin America, Europe, Africa and Asia demonstrate different trajectories of historical and contemporary urbanisation and futures of urban growth. The examples we have brought together from cities in Brazil, UK, China and Africa are distinguished by different histories of colonial power and economic development; different traditions of political systems, ethical settlements and contested urban pasts and presents. These differences of geography and history matter. So while the challenges of urban public health are shared and there is extraordinary potential for cities to learn from each other, the implications of technological change, the capacity to manage mass concentrations of people and the lessons from different experiences of public health interventions are shaped by very different histories and geographies. At any one time the working of the metropolis may privilege particular drivers; the logic of markets, automobile mobilities, public interests defined by the party or a dominant social group, structuring present-day formations that create what complex systems theorists describe as path-dependent historical patterns. Consequently, cities are shaped by particular regimes of property ownership, modes of transport or distributions of power and privilege that generate structural obstacles to optimal health interventions alongside technocratic deployment of new technologies and medical expertise.

We need always to remember the importance of this diversity. In this volume, as our second starting point, we argue that this geographical and historical variation is central to both a plausible sense of policy engagement with urban context and a conceptual framing of how diversity structures the complex systems that link city life to urban health. Cities invariably bring together different systems of resource allocation and culture: economic logics, transport systems, ecological dynamics, normative measures of value and intergenerational obligation. These 'systems of systems' create 'interfaces' between them, demands that can run up against each other, for example in tensions between individuals to exert personal freedoms to maximise the size and shape of their own homes and exercise private property rights versus the logic of city densification that many argue optimises ecological metabolism. Linking public health imperatives to the multiple drivers of city form consequently demands a connection between the understandings of the dilemmas of city commons, the pitfalls and possibilities of intervention, and a conceptual framing of how the city works as an aggregated 'system of systems'.

Empirically, the city is a self-evident form with a complicated, contradictory and sometimes illusory definition. Some urban scholars have spent considerable time theorising the urban. Whether reading the city as a palimpsest, a person or an organism, the subject of the metropolis is itself a chimera (de Souza Santos, 2019). In one reading the globe is overtaken by 'planetary urbanism' (Brenner and Schmid, 2012); in another modernity and the city become indistinguishable (Saunders, 1978). Likewise *public* health is a self-evident subject with a complex and sometimes contradictory definition. The focus on defining the public domain means that a seemingly simple prefix can expand to cross a spectrum of pathologies from forms of collectively measured communicable diseases to multiple aggregated individual acts of knife crime. In this context the attempts to understand how the city itself can be understood as pathogenic has evolved through time.

The global urban turn of the twenty-first century has also increasingly focused interest on the global south, with a proliferation of megacities developing alongside rapid demographic concentration across the urban hierarchy that has resulted in a growing profile of urban public health in development policy internationally. In the mainstream medical domain for the prestige journal *The Lancet* public health is defined by the four elements of decision-making processes based on data, a focus on populations rather than individuals, a goal of social justice and equity, and an emphasis on prevention rather than curative care (Koplan et al., 2009). Each of these four elements is in practice contested across time and between different places globally.

Historically, the legitimacy of city governments in the wake of the industrial revolution was largely rooted in the imperative to create a healthy – or at least inhabitable – city. The interaction of many different systems, networks and forms of organisation that affect the health of residential populations frames the city as an arena in which public health becomes a subject of official concern and a defining logic of governmental intervention. Circulations of air, water, food and energy, the nexus between them and their consolidation in carbon footprint, city metabolism, built environment and lifestyle dispositions have an impact on the longevity and quality of life of urban populations. The industrial cities of nineteenth-century Europe and North America inspired a public concern with the interaction of communicable diseases with sewage and water quality, and provided in some ways both a justification and a defining logic of the modern state rooted in the nineteenth-century metropolis. Imperatives of city governance rationalised a new geography of interventions through state-regulated and frequently state-provided public works in the emergent urban system, defining workplace, home place and the spaces between the two (Osborne and Rose, 1999). The links between the circulations of people and the circulations of the healthy body have likewise structured macro-changes as major as the move to the suburbs and the early garden city planning logics of Ebenezer Howard (Sennett, 1994).

More recently, from the mid-1980s in the north and across the southern urban globe from the 1990s, the growing recognition of the significance of urban context in shaping the effectiveness of medical interventions has been at the heart of the Healthy Cities programmes of the World Health Organization (WHO). The obesity crisis of recent decades prompts debates about the interaction of urban design, personal exercise regimes and public health (Berke et al., 2007). But the connections that join the industrial past and the urban present have constructed both the city itself and the goal of public health in very different ways. The contemporary city context is shaped by the changing economic systems of the last fifty or so years; regimes of economic governance commonly characterised as neoliberal in the global north and its spheres of global influence, the dramatic rise of some middle-income countries in the late twentieth century, particularly in south-east Asia, and the distinctive China model of economic growth and social governance in the twenty-first century. All create contested urban development landscapes in which the logics of public health initiatives must intervene. In an urbanised and connected world, how to design spaces conducive to health gains precedence over what health means across different life prisms, which include culture, gender, class and age.

In this introduction we not only introduce the volume as a whole but also argue that a synthesis of complex systems theory and analysis of common pool resource problems at the heart of urban public health initiatives demands a reconfigured interdisciplinary coalition of scholarship and praxis to think about the interface of the new urban science and the citizens, communities and governments of everyday cities globally. We identify three aspects of this new configuration that structure this introduction:

1. The potential of new sources of real-time 'big data' that grows exponentially our *ability to read urban pattern* but also *qualifies the power of prediction*, enhancing massively a facility to read pattern at scale and individually in the short term while recognizing logically the limits of extrapolating from revealed trends over the longer term.
2. The drivers of *emergence* and recombination in complex systems that generate non-linearity in the urban system and create new urban combinations of culture and nature, infrastructure and humanity, material and behaviour that reconfigure the architecture of public health systems repeatedly disrupted by technological innovations and scientific advances.
3. The imperative to consider how different registers of *value* and *worth* challenge the *commensuration* of different forms of expertise and adopted knowledge in the city. How we reconcile the expertise of social science and natural science surfaces trade-offs between the logics of competing priorities at the heart of different regimes of urban public health.

In the concluding chapter of the volume we go on to consider a fourth dimension of this new configuration. The implications of new urban sciences that engage social scientific and medical knowledges simultaneously demand a new urban imaginary. To consider how they collectively open up different scenarios of the healthy city implies *thinking experimentally* about optimising public health interventions in global processes of urban transformation. Such a disposition consequently also implies a newly engaged form of urban scholarship.

Uncertain futures and complex systems: the value and the limits of prediction

In the nineteenth and twentieth centuries, the escalation of mapping, representations and measurements of the pathologies of city life pluralised understanding of both the numbers of structures that interacted in shaping the health of city residents and the numbers of distal sources of ill health (Olson, 1996). From early studies of inadequate sanitation and poor air quality to the links between the metropolis and mental life and vulnerabilities to communicable diseases, all were rooted back to configurations of urban form. Numerous studies of urban health have followed this tradition over the last century and proliferated in recent decades, cataloguing the determinants of urban health, and at times making a linear and commonly causal connection between urban sites and healthy (or unhealthy) consequences. Much of this scholarship is descriptively powerful, but it too often falls prey to what the literary critic Northrop Frye once described as the fallacy of the scholar 'putting his [sic] favourite study into a causal relationship with whatever interests him less' (Frye, 1957, 6).

Commonly such work identifies patterns that emerge at the interface of two or more urban systems where description becomes powerful but both the aetiology of health outcomes and the causal significance of specific variables become less easily captured in analysis. For example, both historically and intuitively urban housing conditions have been seen as a social cause for concern and are assumed, alleged and in some ways proved to be a cause of major public health challenges. Respiratory diseases, communicable diseases and illnesses of various kinds attributed to poor environment were all clustered in conditions of poor housing, and so across the globe the industrial concentrations of residential poverty in the nineteenth, twentieth and twenty-first centuries have defined sites for public health intervention through housing improvement schemes. But as one historical survey suggests, the causal chains associated with poor housing have become so complex that empirical research generating data informed interventions is constrained because, while some of the first interventions of public health saw the improvement of housing as a fundamental element of tackling poverty, 'the link between housing and the health of the public has become less direct, it has also become more wide-ranging; housing remains a key social determinant of health and (also) a central component of the relationship between poverty and health' (Shaw, 2004: 413).

To exemplify, in East London in the 1990s it was possible to identify houses with large Bangladeshi families living in overcrowded conditions in poor-quality housing stock suffering disproportionate respiratory and communicable disease burden with significant earlier mortality for Bangladeshi men. But precise causally hypothecated and proportionate models were less easily proved. How much of the early mortality rate for Bangladeshi first-generation migrants was attributable to specific housing stock conditions (such as damp, poor insulation and water penetration) and dwelling patterns (such as considerable overcrowding of commonly ten to fifteen people living in two-bedroom flats) as opposed to complex earlier lifestyles in Bangladesh, food poverty, dietary choice, work patterns and expectations and a diverse range of poverty indicators was far less clear. The policy imperative to improve housing conditions was generically self-evident. The extent to which housing policies might be justified on public health grounds, ethical imperatives, political priorities or rational real estate investment, in contrast, was as irrelevant as deciding whether to blame two parts of hydrogen or one part of oxygen in addressing the symptoms of getting wet and catching pneumonia by falling into an East End dock. Equally housing upgrade alone, however, does not change racial or religious prejudices, or unemployment and poverty, which may be determinants of housing choices and ultimately affect access to health systems (Slater, 2013; Gazard et al., 2018). Policy imperatives in this sense may be indifferent to precise and calculable attributions of relative causal significance. But as contemporary data science provides increasingly powerful descriptions of data patterns, there is room to question whether the search for the most powerful or effective public health interventions in emergent cities will return to some core questions about how we make sense of the fundamental notion of causality itself.

In this context, relations in cities between public health and factors as diverse as open space (Brawner et al., 2017; Kondo et al., 2018), exercise (Daumann et al., 2014), police violence (Cooper and Fullilove, 2016), neighbourhood effects and spatial logics (Kwarteng et al., 2017), libraries (Morgan et al., 2017), pest infestation (Shah et al., 2018), food supply (Tach and Amorim, 2015) or race (Tung et al., 2017; Vaughan, Cohen and Han, 2018; Young and Pebley, 2018) are all assiduously mapped, indexed and located in a city space that is pathogenic in a growing science of urban public health. Such research is sophisticated and powerful. But while the data analysis becomes more sophisticated and such scholarship is important, it still at times engages much less with the interdependency of different systems than descriptively with an implicit linearity of singular facets of public health determination.

However, the vast expansion of data generation and the analytical power of data analytics has made it increasingly plausible to analyse in real time the patterns that emerge from a proliferation of sources generated by the contemporary urban environment. Biobank data generating longitudinal measures of sometimes very large numbers of individuals, tracking of behaviours through virtual traces, large-scale experimental data, online footprints of many millions that are frequently geolocated through mobile phone records, consumer expenditure and transaction data, and mobility patterns individualised through identity or travel cards, Google Earth and satellite data can all be subjected to 'big data' analytical tools such as machine learning, image scraping and computational linguistics for the treatment of massive stores of text, video and audio material, producing powerful tools to describe contemporary city life in real time. As much as 95 per cent of such big data is unstructured, leading to an imperative to recognise that the 'heterogeneity, noise, and the massive size of structured big data calls for developing computationally efficient algorithms that may avoid big data pitfalls, such as spurious correlation' (Gandomi and Haider, 2015: 137).

Digital shadows can increasingly be translated into powerful descriptive analysis of public health patterns. The relationship between such patterns and notions of causality is, however, more complicated when confronted by the foundational logic of complex systems theory that starts with the analytical definition of the city as a system of systems driving form and function in the contemporary metropolis. It demands a profoundly important synthesis of both the power of data modelling and the half-life limits of our ability to predict. Pete Allen, a theoretical physicist by background but also one of the most creative thinkers of the way in which such complex systems thinking might unlock the working of cities, has argued that for this reason it is essential to distinguish between the degree to which it is possible to project trend into the future on the basis of modelling and rely on certain forms of system prediction (Allen, 2016). He has made the argument that in complex systems the value of such material diminishes according to the time scales of systemic evolution that form the basis of probabilisitic system dynamics. While models may be used to generalise rank size rules and power laws and even do planning experiments, the innate determinism is qualified by systemic evolution and disruption. Because complex systems are open and not closed they are never stable in the long run. Equilibrium is rarely found in the short run, and never present in the long run. For Allen, forecasting may be valuable in the short run, diminishingly so as systems evolve, simultaneously both valorising and qualifying the quantitative modelling of urban form and pattern. Depending on the pace of systemic evolution, the 'short run' may describe a period of time vulnerable to intervention which may be measured in years, days or hours, and varies enormously between systems. So while it is possible to harness data analytics, model changing urban reality and reveal possible emergent configurations of current structures, Allen argues that models or interpretative frameworks do not make formal *predictions* as such. For him they are instruments of reflection precisely because the mutable form of complex systems makes the inference and attributions of causality ever more challenging. This is particularly important when focusing on bespoke and generalised interventions in urban public health, where the consequences of intervention are always both most immediate in saving lives and most challenging for their (multi-generational) longer-term ethical and legal setting.

Much literature in public health readily acknowledges precisely this challenge (Galea, Riddle and Kaplan, 2010; Diez Roux, 2011; Hammond, 2009). Glass et al (2013) have argued that the problem is particularly pronounced in public health literatures because the inference of causal determinants is rarely straightforward, because the attribution of causality in public health settings is particularly implicated in legal consequences and potential litigation, and because causes are in this sense only those things that could, in principle, be 'treatments' in experiments that may be ethically impossible in real-life settings. They suggest that 'since 1970, the frequency and intensity of formal discourse on causation and causal inference have increased, and the field has progressed toward what we term the modern approach, based on the counterfactual or potential outcomes framework', and so in public policy terms 'the guidelines used to evaluate evidence have not changed for decades, even as the causal questions have become more complex'. As a result they argue that public health policy discussion moves more clearly to a 'potential outcomes framework' because while experimentation city by city might be ideal and randomised control trials would equally provide ideal experimental framing of public health interventions, 'unfortunately, such randomised experiments are often unethical, impractical, or simply too lengthy for timely decision making. As a result, causal inferences for public health are usually derived from observational studies, buttressed by other lines of evidence if available.' They further argue that in public health the connection between spatial pattern and health outcomes constitutes a generic problem in defining causal inference and that 'the utility of long-used, familiar approaches for statistical analysis and causal inference to interpret the broad sweep of evidence on the causal determinants of human health is diminishing' (Glass et al., 2013: 67, 71).

One alternative route out of this dilemma that challenges the configurations of complex systems, policy interventions and public health can also be derived from rethinking the interplay of the biological and the social through a framing that foregrounds public health more in terms of a sense of propensity or *emergence* of patterns in specific contexts. For example, the study of urban mental health has prompted Nikolas Rose and colleagues to return to the theoretical foundations of social science in analysis of the relationship between the metropolis and mental health. In his chapter in this volume, Rose returns to Simmel's foundational framing of the challenge of the modern metropolis and mental health, using contemporary neurological consideration of the location of new epigenetics' recognition of the influence of context in structuring the constitutive transformations between 'the biological' and 'the sociocultural' across the 'life course'. Drawing on the theoretical work of Kurt Goldstein and Georges Canguilhem in a revised vocabulary of vitalism, Nikolas Rose has stressed the imperative of 'seeking to reframe sociological theory to recognise the significance of the biological, and challenging the illusory boundary between the organism and its milieu' (Rose, this volume). In this context, although the city is commonly seen as pathogenic – and at times the chapter treads close to a search for pathological framing – it is also important to recognise that the milieu of the urban, while generating disproportionate challenges of mental health, is also a site of care and sustenance for individuals with severe mental illness.

Rose's contribution forms part of a wider rediscovery of 'vitalism' in the social sciences more generally (e.g. Osborne, 2016; Meloni, Williams and Martin, 2017; Stengers, 2014) as well as bridging social and natural science. Following Canguilhem's injunction that 'A philosophy which looks to science for the clarification of concepts cannot disregard the construction of science', we might, however, take from science studies and the turn to the biosocial in the relatively new academic discipline of Science and Technology Studies (STS) that there may be worries of displacing an old and slightly anachronistic debate between causal notions of mechanism contrasted with sociocultural explanations with a new juxtaposition of mechanism set against a vitalism revivified (Wolfe and Wong, 2014). But perhaps more powerfully, the sense of the vitalists that atmosphere, context and the sociocultural steer away from a simplistic conceptualisation of determinism resonates in a number of philosophical and analytical trends across the boundary territory between social and natural sciences. In part it echoes the realist philosophical distinction that the former professor of the philosophy of science Rom Harré argued for when advocating a stress on the Aristotelian dimensions of the causal; where Aristotle's framing of the material causality of the stone that shaped the formulation of the statue was constitutive of what the statue might become, its sense of possibility was as significant as the formal, efficient and final interventions of the intervention of the sculptor, the axe that shaped the stone and the template against which the statue was modelled. Such a sense of *becoming* is found in much of the more contemporary and in many ways very different genres of social science literature that draws on Deleuzian philosophy, a Latourian notion of the assemblage, and that focuses on the agency of infrastructures and what the China studies expert Francois Jullien references as the Mandarin notion of *shi* or 'the propensity of things' (Jullien, 1995).

This sense of propensity is helpful in considering the historical legacies of city formation, particularly when distinguishing between the time scales of interventions in public health. In this spirit the chapter in this volume by the former deputy mayor of Rio de Janeiro Luiz Eduardo Soares argues that the deep-rooted historical damages of slavery are central to the DNA of the contemporary Brazilian city: they are effectively constitutive of how we make sense of the mental health of the city and can be comprehended only on a long historical canvas. Understanding propensity also dovetails with the sense in which complex systems theory stresses the importance of both the path dependencies of system change and the lock-ins of specific configurations of infrastructure when coming to terms with cities as sociotechnical systems where interfaces within the system between, for example, food systems, water systems and energy systems may change at variable speeds. So the consideration of *speed* as a variable of sociotechnical systems becomes particularly germane when considering the future of the cities that will structure the nature of global urbanism. The divergent patterns in the cities of China, India and Africa in particular and the global south in general will account for the major part of future urban growth, but their speed of growth will inevitably condition the most appropriate public health interventions, potentially raising trade-offs between what is *possible* in the specific geographical and historical contexts of rapid urban growth and what is *ideal* in terms of twenty-first-century sustainable urban form. Urban public health analysis, diagnostic scholarship and optimal policy interventions will consequently need to reflect this diversity, acknowledging challenges that are shared but also how combinations of infrastructure, law, economy, culture and built environment structure urban form distinctively in each emergent metropolis across the global south and north alike. The rhythm and the speed of the possibilities of urban change in different contexts are a constitutive feature of any public policy calculus as much as the propensities of particular combinations of governance, social and material urban forms.

The propensity of infrastructure: city path dependencies, timing, speed and the power of emergence

Technological change recalibrates the optimal spatial configuration of any health system. In the nineteenth century and for much of the twentieth communicable disease was a major killer in the city, optimal primary health care demanded a network of centralised hospitals and dispersed health professionals. And as health research progressed throughout the twentieth century the speed with which it was possible to access particular medical treatments was recognised as key to addressing particular forms of morbidity. This might be measured in terms of geographical distance to primary care hospitals. It might be more immediate and measured in minutes and hours, as with access to public-access defibrillators in the 1990s and early 2000s increasingly deployed in locations with large numbers of people to be used by the general public. It might be measured in days and weeks, as with diagnostic treatment of cancers. So in health terms, speed and space are mutually realised, generating an optimal distribution through space of health resources at any one moment in time. But as technology changes optimal geographical distribution of health infrastructures change likewise.

And the configuration of the built environment is rarely able to change as fast as the optimal distribution of health resources. Like all open systems, cities have *path dependencies* where the history of urban form inhibits some kinds of change and promotes others. Just as technological change restructures the optimal distribution of public health resources, such changes do not take place on a geographical *tabula rasa* but follow on from pre-existing configurations of city life. It is consequently essential to understand the history and context of these path dependencies, the ethnography of technological change, the normative compromises and the trade-offs surfaced by emergent city forms and the institutional logics of city governance through which such change is mediated. 'Seeing like a city' demands a sensibility informed by modelling and analysis generated in the natural sciences, and engagement of the social sciences embedded in particular histories and contingent cultures. It also demands that we find ways of making commensurable the forms of research knowledge generated by different academic disciplinary traditions.

In the United Kingdom (UK) in the late 'noughties' (2000s), much institutional effort and public debate concerned the putative advantages of polyclinics and polysystems, general-practitioner-led health centres that were much promoted in the review of UK National Health Service (NHS) resources (Hutt et al., 2010; NHS, 2008; NHS London, 2010). One of the barely hidden secrets of city life in contemporary Britain has been for some time that a generic model of the 'hospital' inadequately captures the plural forms of primary care and the differentiated optimal accessibilities and centralisations of different medical specialisms. For some medical specialisms it makes sense to centralise regionally, while for others rapid access is more appropriate. The optimal distribution of accident and emergency facilities is different from the optimal distribution of stroke or cancer care. And so the nineteenth-century roots of public health care in the UK and the twenty-first-century imagination of the NHS map uneasily onto this diversity, structured simultaneously by the propensities of both technological advances and built environment infrastructure lock-ins.

In contrast, defibrillators were first invented in the late nineteenth century by the Geneva-based doctors Jean-Louis Prevost and Frederic Batelli, and various medical advances realised their value in situations of cardiac arrest. For many decades defibrillation was used only in hospital, and while some mobile devices were trialled as early as the 1960s in Belfast, it was only in the 1990s in the more affluent parts of the globe that defibrillators were installed in ambulances. And only in the last decade has technological innovation created devices that are cheap enough to be considered for wider use and rapidly proliferated across multiple locations in cities of much of the globe. The reason for this was the combination and trade-offs of city speeds: the speed at which it was possible for the sick to move across the city, the speed that was needed to address cardiac arrest and the speed that it might take to provide public health response to individual cases dispersed across the urban landscape.

According to the British Heart Foundation, the emergency services' average response time to a cardiac-event-related incident in an urban area in the UK is eleven minutes. For every minute that goes by where a victim of sudden cardiac arrest does not receive treatment, their chance of survival decreases by 10 per cent. If defibrillation through a defibrillator occurs within one minute of the victim collapsing, the victim's survival rate increases to 90 per cent. As a result the last decade and a half have seen a massive increase in the deployment of defibrillators in urban settings. Researchers estimated that between 2005 and 2013, the number of defibrillators in Japan went up from just below 11,000 to over 400,000 (Kitamura et al., 2016). Similar exponential growth patterns were found in most cities in Europe and North America.

As a piece of technology the defibrillator reconfigures the optimal provision of public health. As a piece of infrastructure it invokes city speeds. It has certain propensities which interact with systems of both public health and urban mobility. The speed of access to a defibrillator is subject to the mobility patterns of transport in the city. The imperative to access a defibrillator offsets the distance of primary care, but as the city slows down because of congestion the imperative to make low tech-cheap devices available at even more sites grows. And while there are challenges in terms of people's ability or inclination to use the technology when the city is seen as public space, a commons of sorts, such ready access moves the dial of public health and saves lives (Deakin, Anfield and Hodgetts, 2018).

The materiality of infrastructure possesses a propensity of speed which nuances the changing technologies of other aspects of public health. In contrast to the quick-access, quick-turnaround treatments of cardiac arrest, longer term conditions may invoke very different imperatives for intervention, different technologies, different capital values and consequently a different interface between the urban systems, infrastructure and public health. A material object such as a magnetic resonance imaging (MRI) scanner is a highly effective three-dimensional imaging device and demands massive capital investment but is particularly effective in long-term conditions such as cancers or skeletal conditions where the clustering of medical expertise may generate economies of scale and medical knowledge. For the MRI a different trade-off exists between potentially longer distances to travel to the technology and different propensities of speed in the infrastructure itself in terms of the relationship between diagnostic power, positive externalities of clustered medical expertise and considered medical intervention. Such differences vary significantly across national boundaries. In 2017 the UK had the twentieth lowest per capita distribution of MRI scanners in the OECD (Clinical Imaging Board, 2017). And so while such variation points to different priorities and quality of public health care, they also imply a logic that points to an optimal distribution of public health resources across an urban hierarchy which is significantly structured by the propensities and the speeds of infrastructure technologies interfacing with the rationing of finite resources and the logic of expertise clustering within the city.

And yet.

The distribution of health service real estate 'locks in' the distribution of health resources to a pattern that reflects the most recent configuration of bricks and mortar. Changes in real estate generally move at a slower speed than changes in technology. A consensus might be easily reached that a city such as London has too many generic hospitals, but to 'close' a local hospital is politically fissile in a liberal democracy and is invariably subject to grassroots protest. Similarly, shrinking cities across the world suffer with hospitals that are too large for a decreasing population and may lack both doctors and patients, but they linger unchanged because of their political role. Buying and selling health real estate to match any new optimal distribution demands a temporality structured by the speed of systems of land-use planning, development control, commissioning and construction. In a very real sense the speed of technological change commonly runs ahead of the speed of even the most mutable built environment; generating a public health debate that is never perfectly informed and public health policy making that is invariably fighting the last war, configuring for a 'just past' optimal distribution rather than the unforeseeable emergent distribution real estate optimum. In this context, in public policy terms it is in principle possible to model across a number of determining variables at any one moment in time, to analyse the propensities of time and space to reconfigure public resources and to generate both models of the ideal and the trade-offs necessary to settle on calculations of the plausible.

In a growing field of interdisciplinary urban studies, infrastructure in this sense is characterised as possessing agency (Larkin, 2013; Amin and Thrift, 2017), a capacity to shape the emergent city but also to both constrain and facilitate different consequences of identical technological innovations. This cautions against simplistic technocratic understandings of the potential of technological change to shift public health outcomes, implying a recognition of different traditions of governance, geography and history in shaping optimal intervention designs dependent on diverse urban systems. Such diversity also foregrounds both existing settlements of the city and emerging challenges that surface the normative domain on which public health systems are based and into which public health reforms are insinuated.

The right not to have rights? Health systems and valuing the urban commons: commensuration and ethical dilemmas

Healthcare systems normally combine in different configurations of collective demand, state provision, public interests and private behaviours. Their design consequently inevitably invokes normative categories of eligibility, cultural definitions of individualised, familial and neighbourhood responsibility, institutional regimes of welfare and insurance, and public and private fiscal restraints. These categories frame both the rational structuring of city public health systems and infrastructure and the urban domains through which both the systemic inequalities of health outcomes and the registers through which the right to public health in the city are mediated and contested.

Classically, public goods implicitly or explicitly invoke and define the capacity and appropriate times and places when collective needs trump individual liberties. New technologies and emergent city forms continually and iteratively make visible the tensions in such trade-offs. Historical and geographical variations in the regulation of the rights to liberty also highlight the regimes of expertise by which such trade-offs are articulated: specifically the domains of law, politics, economics and constitutional settlement through which value is measured differently and configurations of the public good are determined in relation to property rights, individual freedoms and collective interests. Critical urban studies in general (and some institutions such as UN-Habitat in particular) have drawn on the 'right to the city' as a powerful framework to inform city policy design. But the challenges of metropolitan public health at moments of urban transformation also invoke the critiques in contemporary political theory from both progressive (Douzinas, 2000) and more conservative (Sumption, 2019) positions of rights discourse and highlight the limits of such framing. Indeed in the European Convention on Human Rights most convention rights are qualified and can be suspended when it is necessary in a democratic society for a legitimate purpose such as the prevention of crime, the economic wellbeing of society or – not insignificantly – the protection of public health. The boundaries of rights discourse, when there might be a 'right not to have rights' through such trade-offs between societal imperatives and human rights, can be seen as powerfully articulated in global north and global south alike, reflecting different development ideologies of individual freedoms and very different trajectories of political settlement internationally.

Self-monitoring, individual rights, nudging and actuarial risk
Wearable devices now offer the opportunity to self-monitor quite detailed measures of health: exercise, diet, heartbeat and so on. But what happens when these devices feed through to third parties – either states or corporates managing the health sector? Looking benevolently both the individual and the state can use such data to 'nudge' individuals towards a healthier lifestyle: exercising more, improving diet and thinking more carefully about the appropriate lifestyle choices. But even an ostensibly benign welfare state system may either obscure or make visible the implications of this fine-scale individualised data when aggregated by geographical scale or through the lens of the city or a nation state. To what extent do individuals become responsible for their own conditions of morbidity related to eating, drinking and exercising? How do publicly funded systems prioritise related conditions such as diabetes or obesity? How do locally financed health systems give preference to one patient's needs over others' in systems rationing finite public resources?

But it is also already the case that private insurance companies incentivise self-monitoring through such devices. In the UK one insurance company offers to pay for a £350 Apple iWatch as part of a deal that pays for private insurance and then registers activity data with the company. This may appear innocent until the data collected by the insurance company aggregates data upwards but also personalises such data downwards and translates it into measures of actuarial risk and premium payment levels for the insurance company. In this context actuarial risk becomes not only a rational data form for private insurance but also simultaneously a public concern for regulation of corporate involvement in public health in Rio or Delhi as easily as London or New York.

These are inevitable normative questions generated by technological changes. They are also innately 'city' questions as social and political worlds reorganise themselves around urban form. In the urban context such data is increasingly easy to harvest, and the ethical dilemmas are no less problematic to resolve.

In part such ethically contested urban transformations follow choreographies that map the limits of liberal thought. When should individual freedoms be constrained by collective obligations, and when should states, corporates or communities have the right to know about, to incentivise, to legislate, to nudge and to rule? The public policy dilemmas of liberal democratic logics have long been subject to both communitarian and radical critique. When the logics of liberal freedoms start to dovetail with neoliberal reforms this can become particularly contentious. Michael Sandel (2012) has in this vein famously critiqued when and where price signalling is and is not acceptable. Is it acceptable to fine parents for being late to pick up their children from school, to incentivise walking to schools by pricing proximate parking or to financially penalise workers who are deemed not to be looking as hard for employment or looking after themselves as well as the state believes they should do? How do we measure value in this context, not least when designing systems of public health in emergent cities? Sandel (2012) argues that market logics crowd out alternative measures of value when market-oriented thinking permeates aspects of life traditionally governed by non-market norms; generating new structures of inequality (for those who cannot pay) but also contaminating, devaluing and corrupting alternative registers of value and worth. Institutional legitimacy is hard won and may be subject to devaluation and challenge.

In a public health context it is rarely straightforward ethically to judge when it is acceptable to use techniques of behavioural 'nudging' and when not. A literature exists that considers when and where it is acceptable for nation states to nudge – with or without transparency – free citizens by building on behavioural scholarship that might originate in forms of subtle marketing, whether this involves the NHS in the UK sending reminder mobile phone texts to limit costly 'no shows' in hospital or making 'free riders' feel guilty, or health agencies in 'socialist' and 'capitalist' states alike promoting 'educational' interference in advertising harmful consumer products such as cigarettes or alcohol or introducing pricing or rationing techniques for harmful commodities such as sugar or salt. Hansen, Skov and Skov (2016) argue that in judging these moral questions a 'Rawlsian' publicity principle should apply where the state is allowed a high level of determination of these ethical dilemmas but must be prepared to defend any policy in public. But they also caution that 'relying on Rawls' publicity principle may seem to be an ethically insufficient safeguard. Governments may, and have been willing to, defend many policies publicly that did not hold up to ethical scrutiny' (Hansen, Skov and Skov, 2016: 247). Specifically, liberal freedoms elide with neoliberal reforms when pricing mechanisms regulate values. One British Medical Association (BMA) report highlights the classic study of Richard Titmuss in 1970, which asserts, in invoking the gift relationship, that blood donoation prompted by notions of solidarity, community and moral obligation were both more efficient and morally superior to systems that paid for blood donation (BMA, 2017: 14).

But making price commensurable with a moral calculus is not the only challenge generated by the combination of public health dilemmas, urban transformation and city emergence. The development of artificial intelligence and the growing sophistication of automated domestic and urban systems generates new configurations of old philosophical dilemmas. The undergraduate philosophy trolley problem of whether it is morally acceptable to divert an uncontrolled train to run down a single person deliberately rather than two or three people accidentally standing in its immediate path acquires new dimensions as automated vehicles become more common features of urban mobility. Massachusetts Institute of Technology (MIT) in 2019 hosted a 'moral machine' where visitors to its website were encouraged to submit judgements on generically similar ethical dilemmas of smart and emergent cities.[2] Should automated vehicles run down the wobbling bicycle that may or may not be out of control or the innocent bystander who may have more of a chance of taking evasive action? The permutations are numerous.

In this context the liberal conceit of rights-based languages and the intuitively progressive urban studies invocations of Lefebvre's 'right to the city' find their limits. As with rights discourse more generally we may readily identify with Hannah Arendt's invocation of the right to have rights. However, we also tacitly or at times explicitly acknowledge – though sometimes with less candour – the right not to have rights, in even the most liberal democratic urban formations, when the imperatives of public goods trump individual or collective freedoms. But the ethical dilemmas of exactly when and where this is and is not acceptable are sometimes slightly more challenging than we might think. In the global north attempts to create individual 'autonomy' as the states divest themselves of responsibility for providential futures has grown apace while at the same time, in countries such as South Africa, James

Ferguson (2015) has argued that nascent welfare states emerge through a new progressive politics of distribution that through cash payments and basic income reforms can impact public health issues such as basic food supply and challenge conventional understandings of neoliberal reforms. In other contexts nascent welfare institutionalisation may appear more as an attempt to 'civilise' and 'tame' urban life in cities such as Dar es Salaam, as Joelsson's work demonstrates (2020). The argument here is not to advocate simple answers to complex questions but to highlight the trade-offs and uncertain futures that may inform attempts to reshape the domain of public health in emergent urban configurations which have to deal with a history of the present and a geography of colonial and other legacies that structure the DNA of some of the most rapidly growing cities in the world, as examples from both China and India can be seen to exemplify.

Trade-offs between economy, rights, freedoms and health provision in the cities of China

Urban health systems are mediated by the twenty-first-century scale of planetary urbanisation that is witnessed globally and commonly narrated through a universal vocabulary. But it is in China and India where the speed and scale of this urban transformation are most pronounced. These two nations alone will account for a significant proportion of global urban growth, and it in this context that the particular trajectories of public health changes in the two countries are of particular interest.

In China in the Mao era regime, legitimacy and public trust focused in part on mass provision of generic hospitals rather than local health clinics, and was also tied historically and logically to post-1948 state provision defining geographically restricted local *hukou* registration. One consequence of the rural bias of Mao's development model, the *hukou* served as a form of 'local citizenship', prescribing access to welfare provision, including health care tied to the combination of home place and workplace in the city *danwei*. In the booming cities of late twentieth-century China in the reform processes triggered by the Deng regime and running from the early 1980s to the present day, the *hukou* system created cities with 'floating populations' who may live in Shanghai, Beijing or Shenzhen but whose health access is determined by hometown *hukou* and hometown local health welfare systems in Szechuan or Xinjiang. And as the economy 'opened up' in the 1980s and public expenditure on health care diminished, individual 'freedoms' 'allowed' people in China increasingly to spend more on their own health care. They consequently saved more providentially, in anticipation of ill fortune. By 1988 individual expenditure on health care exceeded state expenditure, and this trend and the consequent differential between the condition of the welfare net and the imperative to increase personal savings accelerated over the following decade. But when people save more they spend less and local demand is reduced, with direct consequences for economic growth. One standard argument based on economic 'values' suggests that 'pooled risk' through strong welfare provision is more likely to enhance consumer demand because families will save less for their own health provision. So while urban welfare provision may appear self-evidently both a normative problem and a social and political challenge, it undoubtedly has strong economic implications. The capacity of urban China to develop beyond the impressive data, moving from low-income to middle-income status for large numbers, may be limited by the consequent lower levels of private expenditure and domestic demand for goods and services and the commensurately higher levels of personal savings that anticipate personal provision for the misfortunes of ill health and unemployment.

In part, following a logic that in this sense is both economic and ethical, this trend was reversed in China from 2001 until by 2014 state expenditure on health care had again overtaken private expenditure (Liu, Vortherms and Hong, 2017: 433; Figure 1.1). More recently still, Xi Jinping has accelerated reforms of the *hukou* system to rationalise urban welfare regimes and reduce the gap between those who hold 'urban citizenship rights' through city-based *hukou* and migrants to the city, although the pace of migration to the cities generally exceeds the pace of *hukou* reform, generating ongoing distinctions between rural to urban migrants and urban 'citizens' (Wu, 2016). But the logic driving the changes was not economic alone. When development reached the point where the health burden switched from communicable to chronic diseases – in China as elsewhere – the logics of the health infrastructure changed likewise, and the need for a dominant network of primary care hospitals was reshaped by imperatives that were no different from those in the liberal democratic global north.

Three kinds of health insurance were introduced by Xi. One was for rural residents, and two were for urban residents: one for those with city *hukou* and one for those without. The former was much better funded

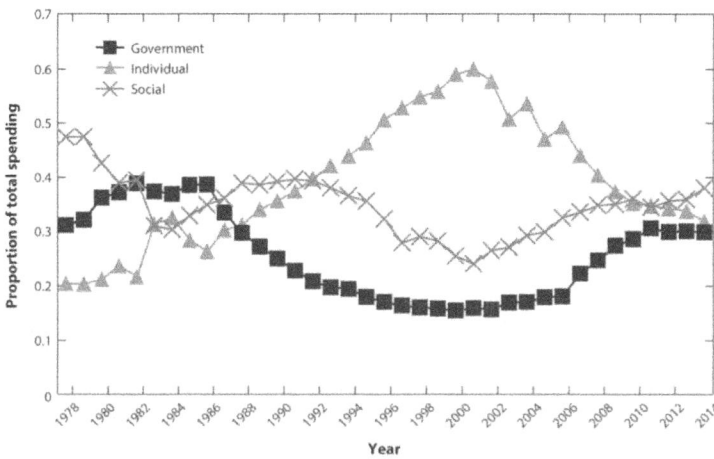

Figure 1.1 Share of total health expenditures (China). From Liu, Vortherms and Hong, 2017: 433. CC-BY-SA 4.0

than the latter. A massive increase in insurance coverage nationally went from below 10 per cent of the population in 1992 to 95 per cent by 2017 (Yue et al, 2017). Yet as a result of the last decade of reform a demographic divide is built into the DNA of the city. For Liu, Vortherms and Hong (2017: 435–6) 'while poorer and more rural areas saw significant improvements in medical insurance coverage, urban areas and wealthier families continue to benefit disproportionately from insurance subsidies because urban insurance plans provide substantively more coverage'.

Wicked problems and 'southern urbanism'

A World Bank water and sanitation project report in 2011 estimated the economic impact of poor water sanitation in India to be equivalent to 6.4 per cent of GDP (World Bank, 2011: 9). With problems worse in the smaller cities than in the larger cities, there are both dire consequences of such patterns in direct impact and the opportunity to leapfrog the particular lock-ins and failures of many northern systems where high-quality sanitised water is piped to houses that do not separate 'brown' from other water and waste; this is significant when in India in 2015 only 35 per cent of human waste was disposed of through piped sewer systems (Jana et al., 2015). But this potential also needs to be set in the context of what Bhan (2019) has described as the constitutive southern urban practices that emerge from the particular emergent urbanisms of India's colonial legacies, constitutional formation and specific forms of inequality, exclusion and consequent social movements. In the conclusion of this volume we draw in more detail on Bhan's exemplification of speedily constructed health centres in Delhi that exploit the ambiguities of Delhi property rights to 'squat' on pavements.

In this context Bhan (2019), in his work addressing the emergent urbanisms of contemporary India, has argued persuasively that an understanding of the DNA of urban life in Delhi depends on decoding the path dependencies and lock-ins that distinguish the practices of 'southern urbanism' as foundational in this regard. He describes the pragmatically successful 'mohalla' health clinics in Delhi. Many of these have transgressed state laws and conventional property rights but are in their own terms a major success. They are in many ways ecologically suboptimal but situationally transformative examples of public health intervention, placing the right to public health over alternative demands on land use within the city, a pragmatism we return to in this volume.

And so when we begin to understand propensity as a framing of causality in terms of both capacities and temporalities, then material infrastructure exhibits not only a 'social life of things' but, as we see with defibrillators in the global north, also an agency of its own. Material configurations affect the evolution of urban systems through their innate properties, their relational setting and their implicit relationship to cartographies and temporalities of the city. In this sense infrastructures assume both a politics and a poetics as well as having the power to generate urban change, a sense of the agency of infrastructure (Appadurai, 1988; Gartner, 2014; Larkin, 2013; Simone, 2019).

In this sense we are arguing gently – and perhaps paradoxically – in the volume that the distinction between an urban studies of the global north and the global south is powerful in some contexts but also can limit understanding of the dynamics of city life globally. Cultural traffic now flows across new geographies and geometries, and city learning might do so likewise, challenging the routed historical export of technocratic solutions from corporates and scholars, primarily in the global north, to cities and communities where problems defined and preferred futures might draw on different shorter- and longer-term answers to urban transformation. In this context, chapters of this volume draw on examples across these cartographies.

Book outline

In Chapter 2 ('Mental health, stress and the contemporary metropolis'), Nikolas Rose returns to one of the founding questions in Simmel's urban studies when considering the interplay of the metropolis and mental health. Rose argues for a recombination of natural sciences and social science expertise in making sense of public health in the city. After initial case studies in Rio, London and São Paulo, he offers a fine-grained analysis of mental health in the contemporary metropolis. While it is hardly surprising that urban life is connected to mental disorder in a context of racism (Chapter 8), gendered violence (Chapter 3) or poor mobility (Chapter 4), there remains the paradox of improved access to better-paid jobs in cities and the presence of community-led initiatives in those areas. Aware of such caveats, Rose also discusses urban perils and their buffers. The key question is how to create mechanisms that understand socially and biomedically how the experience of poverty, inequality, racism or gender discrimination may lead to mental distress. Such a mechanism, Rose sustains, is key to avoiding misidentification of key roots in the provision of wellbeing. In a society yearning for life quality, all too often simplified explanations may create short-lived solutions, such as when simply changing housing conditions is expected to improve mental health. However, a more holistic mechanism of analysis would look at remaining mental distress from past experiences and consider the causes that led people to live in poor housing conditions in the first place (Slater, 2013). Thus, the creation of healthy, safe or sustainable cities may include discussing a new biopolitics that uses both ethnography and urban studies to address spatial, sensorial and temporal characteristics of stress. While geomapping apps may already link distress with particular areas of the city, what such apps cannot see is how people search for help, often outside official medical services. With a normative conclusion, Rose epitomises the need to understand 'capabilities that are required to lead a fulfilled life', which will require restructuring mental health services, looking especially at the viewpoint of those who are users and not providers of health services.

In the last decade the World Health Organization has suggested that violence against women is a major global health priority, and McIlwaine et al. in Chapter 3 ('Feminised urban futures, healthy cities and violence against women and girls: transnational reflections from

Brazilians in London and Maré, Rio de Janeiro') draw on this expanded consideration of public health to discuss the incidence of transnational violence against women and girls. Looking at cities as places where violence against women occurs in the public and private realms, as well as places where women can access better-paid jobs, potentially leading to self-development, the authors discuss the urban paradox regarding women's health and wellbeing, focusing on Rio de Janeiro and London. This chapter is linked to other work on Brazil in this volume by addressing domestic violence and gender-based violence, both often overlooked in places such as Rio, which, as Luiz Eduardo Soares explains, have high incidences of male homicide rates. How do women navigate the city? How does gender-based violence affect health? How is income obstructed by events of violence? Finally, how do women perceive events of physical, psychological and financial violence, and which mechanisms do they have to respond? The authors answer those questions, combining theories on gendered cities and urban violence with life stories. In Rio, the research took place in Maré, a favela complex in the north of the city where public spaces can be a site of violence. In London, working and domestic spaces are key risky environments. A central discussion in the chapter shows how violence travels by epitomising the stories of migrant women trying to escape violence and yet being victims once again. Patriarchal structures are indeed entrenched in Brazil and the UK, even if they are manifested differently. By finishing with a discussion of what safety is and what it entails in the city, with a focus on livelihoods access and the ability to participate in every aspect of public life, the chapter contributes to a broader discussion of how we can understand the urban in its private and public realms and gendered perspectives, as well as how language and access to support networks impact wellbeing and urban health.

Adding to this complex discussion of how a city can be experienced differently according to race (Soares) or gender (McIlawaine et al.), Schwanen and Nixon in Chapter 4 ('Understanding the relationships between wellbeing and mobility in the unequal city: the case of community initiatives promoting cycling and walking in São Paulo and London') discuss the intersectional spaces between domestic and public spheres, looking at spaces of mobility. They identify our lack of standardised measures of wellbeing, arguing for the importance of the link between urbanisation and a more nuanced definition of wellbeing. The authors put everyday mobility at the centre of their analysis, because for them wellbeing and mobility are concepts situated in time-spaces and therefore 'always differentiated and differentiating'. When exploring the wellbeing-mobility nexus in London and São Paulo, the authors demonstrate that in both cities navigating urban spaces can be a barrier to experiencing happiness. Interviews with cyclists in these two cities show how community-led initiatives are filling gaps left by the state in the provision of transport. In São Paulo, for example, while public transport may be available, there are spaces that are considered unsafe and out of reach despite existing routes. Thus integrating spaces is also about providing safety in those areas. Group walks, by diminishing fear of crime, may also reduce journey distances by opening up more direct routes through areas previously regarded as unsafe. Equally, bicycle repair shops may be gender- and class-biased territories, and community-led initiatives have addressed the problem by making bicycle repairs available to disadvantaged groups. Citizen-led initiatives show how cycling and walking can affect wellbeing.

Chapter 5, 'Urban (sanitation) transformation in China: a Toilet Revolution and its socio-eco-technical entanglements', also advocates a systemic approach (socio-eco-technical) to address sanitation in its social, material, economic and cultural interfaces, because 'Sanitation is shaped by and shapes culture, identity and representation; equally, it is interlinked with economic processes across a multitude of scales'. Regarding toilets as a lens through which to discuss the fast-paced urbanisation of China and its multidimensional consequences, Deljana Iossifova stresses the importance of combining economic and cultural processes to address and theorise cities. She does so by discussing the use of flushing toilets in China as a symbol of development and simultaneously as an instrument of intergenerational distancing and a medium to enhance existing economic difference. A response to the provision of sanitation in cities thus needs to address ecological, material, economic, cultural and political aspects, without running the risk of a one-size-fits-all idea that flushing toilets can be a preferred solution in all contexts. Instead, the author favours provincialised responses to sanitation demands as a way to tackle culture, identity and representation, and not only economical and ecological processes.

Ecological, material, economic and political aspects of sanitation also feature in Warren Smit's discussion of the food environment and health in African cities in Chapter 6, 'The food environment and health in African cities: analysing the linkages and exploring possibilities for improving health and wellbeing'. Food environments are discussed, considering factors that have an impact on the production, retail and consumption of food in cities. Looking at African cities, where food insecurity is high, Smit discusses food outlets in cities – most of them 'at the informal end of the formality–informality continuum', where infrastructure, shelter and transport, as well as urban agriculture, address both the availability and the affordability of food. Poor transport, for example, might make local products more expensive than imported goods, and thus to understand food security, it is fundamental to illuminate the nexus connecting infrastructure and governance with the ability to store, prepare, transport and consume food as well as dispose of its waste. The author argues that environments that are conducive to food security are those that allow for land-use zoning, the provision of infrastructure (water, sanitation, energy, transport) and the improvement of governance of food systems. On the aspect of governance, agreeing with Iossifova, he upholds that decentralised governance is helpful for addressing infrastructure challenges. Finally, Smit supports transdisciplinary research on food environments as a way forward to see the food environment as a complex system that crosses disciplines as well as government sectors.

After a succession of chapters that have discussed cities around the globe, Chapter 7 addresses different neighbourhoods within the same city. In 'Urban mental health and the moral economies of suffering in a "broken city": reinventing depression among Rio de Janeiro urban dwellers', Leandro David Wenceslau and Francisco Ortega discuss urban mental health through the perspective of both health practitioners and health users in Rio's affluent ('asphalt') and poor ('hill') locations. This chapter shows that while wealthy residents are more likely to look for and access official mental health services, the poor, when they search for mental health services, do so in more critical situations. When addressing social, cultural, moral and material conditions that influence the search for mental health professionals and the interactions between medical doctor and patient, the authors also offer a reading of Rio's recent context of economic decline, which has led to a fall in life quality among middle-class residents. Those residents who used to have access to private health facilities, well-paid jobs and other conveniences in the city are likely to search for mental health support when facing unemployment or worse employment situations, while the poor may be more used to intense and continuous disruption in housing or employment situations, which the authors discuss as a form of mental health resilience in times of economic decline.

The final chapter is prefaced by a short introduction of the author – Luiz Eduardo Soares – an academic anthropologist who also played a senior mayoral role in the metropolis of Rio de Janeiro during the Lula regime and then also served as the National Secretary of Public Security. He characterises Rio de Janeiro as an exaggerated version of Brazil and, for that reason, an ideal place to observe the causes and effects of violence in everyday life. To begin, the author alerts any hasty scholar that the exaggerated rates of violence in the city should not give the false impression that the problem is ubiquitous. Soares explains the prevalence of violence among young, black and poor favela residents. Looking at wellbeing in the city of Rio thus requires understanding historical socio-spatial segregations. From slavery to drug policies, this chapter explains how historical political decisions have scarred a society over time. Fighting clichés of Brazil as a place of indiscriminate violence and impunity, the chapter addresses the predominance of incarceration among those who are also more likely to be victims of violence. The poor in Rio as victims of all sorts of violence are a prism through which one can see racism as the predominant imperative that formed Brazilian society, with violence as the language that maintains such order.

In what follows, the chapters explore health and mental health across different cities in Brazil, China, the UK and South Africa, demonstrating that to understand wellbeing in cities entails a fundamental conversation about race, gender, mobility, food systems and economic systems, and that we need to expand how we measure wellbeing. A focus on users of health systems and ethnographic approaches drawn from the social sciences gain centrality in a new biopolitics of the emerging city alongside the powerful analytical domains of the new urban sciences.

Acknowledgements

This book was completed with support from the ESRC Urban Transformations Programme and also from PEAK Urban programme, funded by UKRI's Global Challenge Research Fund, Grant Reference: ES/P011055/1.

Notes

1 The final drafts of this volume were completed just before the COVID-19 pandemic first became visible in Wuhan in China in late 2019. While the pandemic is not addressed at all in the collection, we believe the issues it addresses are of pressing concern, not least how we consider the city as both a commons and a complex system at a time of public health crisis.
2 See MIT Moral Machine, http://moralmachine.mit.edu (last accessed 1 November 2019).

References

Allen, P. (2016). The co-evolving complexity of cities: Towards sustainability. DACAS Summer School, Manchester, online video, www.complexurban.com/video/183/ (last accessed 1 November 2019).

Amin, A., and Thrift, N. (2017). *Seeing like a city*. Cambridge and Malden, MA: Polity Press.

Appadurai, A. (1988). *The social life of things: Commodities in cultural perspective*. Cambridge: Cambridge University Press.

Berge, E., Cole, D.H., and Ostrom, E. (eds) (2012). *Property in land and other resources*. Cambridge, MA: Lincoln Institute of Land Policy.

Berke, E.M., Koepsell, T.D., Moudon, A.V., Hoskins, R.E., and Larson, E.B. (2007). Association of the built environment with physical activity and obesity in older persons. *American Journal of Public Health*, 97(3): 486–92.

Berkes, F. (2017). Environmental governance for the Anthropocene? Social-ecological systems, resilience, and collaborative learning. *Sustainability*, 9(7), art. 1232.

Bhan, G. (2019). Notes on a Southern urban practice. *Environment and Urbanization*, 31(2): 1–19.

BMA (2017). The ethical implications of the use of market-type mechanisms in the delivery of NHS care. London: British Medical Association.

Brawner, B.M., Guthrie, B., Stevens, R., Taylor, L., Eberhart, M., and Schensul, J.J. (2017). Place still matters: Racial/ethnic and geographic disparities in HIV transmission and disease burden. *Journal of Urban Health*, 94(5): 716–29.

Brenner, N., and Schmid, C. (2012). Planetary urbanization. In M. Gandy (ed.), *Urban constellations*, 10–13. Berlin: Jovis.

Clinical Imaging Board (2017). Magnetic resonance imaging (MRI) equipment, operations and planning in the NHS Royal College of Radiologists. London: Clinical Imaging Board.

Colding, J., and Barthel S. (2019). Exploring the social-ecological systems discourse 20 years later. *Ecology and Society*, 24(1), art. 2.

Cooper, H.L.F., and Fullilove, M. (2016). Editorial: Excessive police violence as a public health issue. *Journal of Urban Health*, 93(1): 1–7.
Daumann, F., Heinze, R., Römmelt, B., and Wunderlich, A. (2015). An active city approach for urban development: Open space and urban health determinants. *Journal of Urban Health: Bulletin of the New York Academy of Medicine*, 92(2): 217–29.
Deakin, C.D., Anfield, S., and Hodgetts, G.A. (2018). Underutilisation of public access defibrillation is related to retrieval distance and time-dependent availability. *Heart*, 104(16): 1339–43.
De Souza Santos, A.A. (2019). *The politics of memory: Urban cultural heritage in Brazil*. London: Rowman and Littlefield.
Diez Roux, A.V. (2011). Complex systems thinking and current impasses in health disparities research. *American Journal of Public Health*, 101(9): 1627–34.
Douzinas, C. (2000). *The end of human rights: Critical legal thought at the turn of the century*. London: Hart Publishing.
Ferguson, J. (2015). *Give a man a fish: Reflections on the new politics of distribution*. London: Duke University Press.
Foster, S.R., and Iaione, C. (2016). The city as a commons. *Yale Law and Policy Review*, 34: 281–349.
Frye, N. (1957). *Anatomy of criticism: Four essays*. Princeton: Princeton University Press.
Galea, S., Riddle, M., and Kaplan, G.A. (2010). Causal thinking and complex system approaches in epidemiology. *International Journal of Epidemiology*, 39(1): 97–106.
Gandomi, A., and Haider, M. (2015). Beyond the hype: Big data concepts, methods, and analytics. *International Journal of Information Management*, 35(2): 137–44.
Gartner, C.M. (2014). *The agency of infrastructure: A critical acquisition framework for understanding infrastructure development within inequitable societies*. Waterloo: UWSpace.
Gazard, B., Chui, Z., Harber-Aschan, L., MacCrimmon, S., Bakolis, I., Rimes, K., Hotopf, M., and Hatch, S.L. (2018). Barrier or stressor? The role of discrimination experiences in health service use. *BMC Public Health*, 18(1), art. 1354.
Glass, T.A., Goodman, S.N., Hernán, M.A., and Samet, J.M. (2013). Causal inference in public health. *Annual Review of Public Health*, 34(1): 61–75.
Hammond, R.A. (2009). Complex systems modeling for obesity research. *Preventing Chronic Disease*, 6(3): A97–A97.
Hansen, P.G., Skov, L.R., and Skov, K.L. (2016). Making healthy choices easier: Regulation versus nudging. *Annual Review of Public Health*, 37(1): 237–51.
Hardin, G. (1968). The tragedy of the commons. *Science*, 162(3859): 1243–48.

Hardt, M., and Negri, A. (2009). *Commonwealth*. Cambridge, MA: Harvard University Press.

Huron, A. (2015). Working with strangers in saturated space: Reclaiming and maintaining the urban commons. *Antipode*, 47(4): 963–79.

Hutt, P., Surinder, S., Modell, M., and Nazareth, I. (2010). Polyclinics and polysystems: Evolving ambiguity, evidence required. *British Journal of General Practice*, 60(575): 400–1.

Jana, A., Malladi, T., Anand, G., Wankhade, K., Vishnu, M.J., Raju, M.J.S., and Rao, P. (2015). Urban water supply and sanitation. In A. Revi (ed.), *Urban India 2015: Evidence*, 93–115. Bangalore: IIHS.

Joelsson, I. (2020). Risky urban futures: the bridge, the fund and insurance in Dar es Salaam. In M. Keith and A. A. de Souza Santos (eds.), *African cities and collaborative futures: urban platforms and metropolitan logistics*. Manchester: Manchester University Press.

Kitamura, T., Kiyohara, K., Sakai, T., Matsuyama, T., Hatakeyama, T. Shimamoto, Izawa, J., Fujii, T., Nishiyama, C., Kawamura, T., and Iwami, T. (2016). Public-access defibrillation and out-of-hospital cardiac arrest in Japan. *New England Journal of Medicine*, 375(17): 1649–59.

Kondo, M. C., Fluehr, J., McKeon, T., and Branas, C. (2018). Urban green space and its impact on human health. *International Journal of Environmental Research in Public Health*, 15(445): 1–28.

Koplan, J., Bond, C., Merson, M., Reddy, S., Rodriguez, M., Sewankambo, N., and Wasserheit, J. (2009). Towards a common definition of global health. *Lancet*, 373: 1993–95.

Kwarteng, J. L., Schulz, A.J., Mentz, G.B., Israel, B.A., and Perkins, D.W. (2017). Independent effects of neighborhood poverty and psychosocial stress on obesity over time. *Journal of Urban Health*, 94(6): 791–802.

Larkin, B. (2013). The politics and poetics of infrastructure. *Annual Review of Anthropology*, 42(1): 327–43.

Liu, G. G., Vortherms, S.A., and Hong, X. (2017). China's health reform update. *Annual Review of Public Health*, 38(1): 431–48.

Meloni, M., Williams, S., and Martin P. (2017). The biosocial: Sociological themes and issues. *The Sociological Review*, 64(1): 7–25.

Morgan, A., Dupuis, R., Davenport-Whiteman, E., D'Alonzo, B., and Cannuscio, C. (2017). Our doors are open to everybody. *Journal of Urban Health*, 94: 1–3.

NHS (2008). *High quality care for all: NHS next stage review*. UK: NHS.

NHS (2010). *Delivering healthcare for London: An integrated strategic plan 2010–2015*. London: NHS.

Olson, D. R. (1996). *The world on paper: The conceptual and cognitive implications of writing and reading*. Cambridge: Cambridge University Press.

Olson, M., Jr. (1965). *The logic of collective action: public goods and the theory of groups.* Cambridge, MA: Harvard University Press.

Osborne, T. (2016). Vitalism as pathos. *Biosemiotics,* 9(2): 185–205.

Osborne, T., and Rose, N. (1999). Governing cities: Notes on the spatialisation of virtue. *Environment and Planning D: Society and Space,* 7: 737–60.

Ostrom, E., Dietz, T., Dolsal, P., Stern, S.S., and Weber, E.U. (eds) (2002). *The drama of the commons.* Washington, DC: National Academies Press.

Sandel, M.J. (2012). *What money can't buy: The moral limits of markets.* New York: Farrar, Straus and Giroux.

Saunders, P. (1978). *Social theory and the urban question.* London: Hutchinson.

Sennett, R. (1994). *Flesh and stone: The body and the city in Western civilization.* New York: W.W. Norton.

Shah, S.N., Fossa, A., Steiner, A.S., Kane, J., Levy, J.I., Adamkiewicz, G., Bennett-Fripp, W.M., and Reid, M. (2018). Housing quality and mental health: The association between pest infestation and depressive symptoms among public housing residents. *Journal of Urban Health,* 95: 691–702.

Shaw, M. (2004). Housing and public health. *Annual Review of Public Health,* 25(1): 397–418.

Simone, A. (2019). *Improvised lives: Rhythms of endurance in an urban south (after the postcolonial).* London: Polity Press.

Slater, T. (2013). Your life chances affect where you live: A critique of the 'cottage industry' of neighbourhood effects research. *International Journal of Urban and Regional Research,* 37(2): 367–87.

Stengers, I. (2014). *Thinking with Whitehead: A free and wild creation of concepts.* Cambridge, MA: Harvard University Press.

Sumption, J. (2019). Human rights and wrongs. Lecture 3 of the 2019 Reith Lectures, BBC, www.bbc.co.uk/programmes/m0005msd (last accessed 1 November 2019).

Tach, L., and M. Amorim (2015). Constrained, convenient, and symbolic consumption: Neighborhood food environments and economic coping strategies among the urban poor. *Journal of Urban Health,* 92(5): 815–34.

Tung, E.L., Cagney, K.A., Peek, M.E., and Chin, M.H. (2017). Spatial context and health inequity: Reconfiguring race, place, and poverty. *Journal of Urban Health,* 94(6): 757–63.

Vaughan, C.A., Cohen, D.A., and Han, B. (2018). How do racial/ethnic groups differ in their use of neighborhood parks? Findings from the National Study of Neighborhood Parks. *Journal of Urban Health,* 95(5): 739–49.

Wilson, J. (2002). Scientific uncertainty, complex systems, and the design of common-pool institutions. In E. Ostrom, T. Dietz, P. Dolsal, S.S. Stern, and E.U. Weber (eds), *The drama of the commons,* 327–36. Washington, DC: National Academies Press.

Wolfe, C.T., and Wong, A. (2014) The return of vitalism: Canguilhem, Bergson and the project of a biophilosophy. In M. De Beistegui, G. Bianco and M. Gracieuse (eds), *The care of life: Transdisciplinary perspectives in bioethics and biopolitics*, 63–75. London and New York: Rowman & Littlefield.

World Bank (2011). *Economic impacts of inadequate sanitation in India*. Washington, DC: World Bank.

Wu, F. (2016). Emerging Chinese cities: Implications for global urban studies. *Professional Geographer*, 68(2): 338–48.

Young, M.T., and Pebley, A.R. (2017). Legal status, time in the USA, and the well-being of Latinos in Los Angeles. *Journal of Urban Health*, 94(6): 764–75.

Yue, D., Ruan, S., Xu, J., Zhu, W., Zhang, L., Cheng, G., and Meng, Q. (2017). Impact of the China Healthy Cities Initiative on urban environment. *Journal of Urban Health*, 94(2): 149–57.

2

Mental health, stress and the contemporary metropolis

Nikolas Rose

Can contemporary developments in the life sciences help us understand the ways in which 'adversity' shapes mental health conditions in the heterogeneous conglomerations we call cities? Many have pointed to the evidence that those living in cities are more likely to be diagnosed with mild, moderate and severe mental disorders than those living in rural settings. But it has proved difficult to identify precisely what it is in the urban experience that leads to these elevated rates. The same is true of research that has addressed urban mental health in migrant and refugee populations, in the global north and in megacities such as Mumbai, Shanghai and São Paulo in the global south. Some rates are elevated in some migrants, sometimes only in the second generation, but the findings are equivocal, and migration itself does not seem to be a consistent causal factor for mental ill health – indeed sometimes quite the reverse.

Can we link biomedical explanations with sociological and anthropological research to understand the ways in which the experiences of poverty, inequality, precarity, gender discrimination, racism, stigma, social exclusion, isolation, threat and violence lead many to mental distress? Can we extend such an analysis beyond these traditional 'social factors' to encompass such issues as the built environment, the capacities and limits to individual and collective life engendered by the urban infrastructure, and the urban 'sensorium' of noise, smell, touch and microbes? If we understood these mechanisms better would we be better able to advise on policies to mitigate mental distress in urban environments and on practices likely to promote recovery? Could such an approach inform strategies to create 'healthy, safe and sustainable cities'[1] through measures ranging from architecture and urban design, through housing, transport and mobilities, to the management of biophysical environments from microbes to air quality? Could we 'translate' such biosocial and biocultural research to policies and practices, and if so, how would questions such as urban justice or the 'right to the city' be transformed? Could we draw upon our genealogical grasp of urban biopolitics to shape another biopolitics of the urban? To paraphrase Didier Fassin (Fassin, 2009), is another politics of life possible?

These are the questions that my research group is addressing in our programme of research on 'The Urban Brain'.[2] This research programme was initiated in 2013 with a grant from the Transformative Research Scheme of the Economic and Social Research Council (ESRC), which enabled us to hold four international workshops and develop the framework for international collaborations around the theme of mental health, migration and the megacity. The first substantive research project focuses on rural-to-urban migration in Shanghai, where we are working with partners from the Department of Public Health at Fudan University on a three-year study funded from the ESRC's Newton Fund. We are using the case of São Paulo, which has a very different pattern and temporality of migration, as a comparator, working with colleagues from the Department of Psychiatry at University of São Paulo Medical School, and are working with colleagues at the Wellesley Institute in Toronto to explore the implications of the very different patterns of migration in Toronto. We are fortunate that, at King's College London, we are also able to make comparisons with the results from the South East London Community Health (SELCoH) study, carried out in the south London boroughs of Southwark and Lambeth, both of which have very large populations of transnational migrants.[3] These experimental empirical investigations explore the mental and cerebral consequences of two of the central transformations that characterise our present – urbanisation and migration.

Reasons to be cheerful, one, two, three, four, five

Our 'urban brain' experiments start from five 'reasons to be (cautiously) cheerful', as follows.[4]

First, there are developments in the life sciences and neuroscience that recognise the limits of the paradigm of social research that has dominated for the last fifty years (disussed in detail in Rose and Abi-Rached, 2013;

Rose and Abi-Rached, 2014). This is leading to a gradual transformation of styles of thought, away from molecular reductionism, with its focus on experiments on animal models in laboratories or isolated individuals in brain scanners, towards approaches that try to relocate the human animal in its milieu, and to a recognition of the constitutive transformations between 'the biological' and 'the sociocultural' across the 'life course'. The words are becoming familiar. Epigenetics, the processes of gene activation and de-activation across an individual's life, in response to inputs from the milieu. Neuroplasticity, the fact that neural circuits are shaped and reconfigured across the life course, both in terms of structure and in terms of function in response to experiences. Neurogenesis, the production and integration of new nerve cells, to replace those that are dead or damaged, a process which can be stimulated or inhibited by factors from exercise to diet. The microbiome, the millions of bacteria which inhabit human and other animals and play an important part in maintaining both physical and mental health, and which are acutely sensitive to the environment and form of life of the human being that they live with. The exposome, the cumulative effect on the organism of environmental insults from pollution and radiation to diet and noise. We may already be bored with the cliché 'how adversity gets under the skin', but social scientists should embrace these developments, not least because the conceptions of the social, the cultural and indeed of 'adversity' in such emerging styles of thought are both etiolated and imprecise.

Second, some social scientists now recognise that not all references to the biological are reductionist, determinist, fatalist and so forth. Humans are indeed biosociocultural creatures, whose capacities, forms of life and life course are not merely discursively enabled and performed, but are shaped in fundamental ways by the fact that they are evolved living creatures, evolved for language, sociality, culture. Pioneers in this regard – Elizabeth Grosz, Elizabeth Wilson and Margaret Lock, and in another way, Ted Benton – are no longer isolated voices (Grosz, 1994; Wilson, 2015; Lock and Kaufert, 2001; Benton, 1993). We now have multiple manifestoes rediscovering the biological roots of the social sciences, seeking to reframe sociological theory to recognise the significance of the biological and challenging the illusory boundary between the organism and its milieu (e.g. Meloni, Williams and Martin, 2016). We should welcome this 'entente cordiale' between the two sciences of life. But we have few studies of specific problems that embody this ethos, and few attempts to link this recognition of the biosociocultural character of human societies with the central questions of the contemporary social sciences concerning power, inequality and injustice.

Third, when it comes to mental health, there is increasing recognition of the role of 'social determinants'. We can see this in the recent report written for the World Health Organization (WHO) by Michael Marmot and his group on 'the social determinants of mental health' (WHO, 2014), and, tentatively, in recent publications by psychologists and psychiatrists, such as the recent report of the Lancet Commission on 'The Future of Psychiatry' (Bhugra et al., 2017). The WHO report is clearest, pointing to systematic reviews that consistently show that common mental disorders such as depression and anxiety 'are distributed according to a gradient of economic disadvantage across society': the poor and disadvantaged suffer disproportionally from common mental disorders and their adverse consequences (Campion et al., 2013; Lund et al., 2010; WHO, 2014), both in low-resource settings (Patel et al., 2010; Patel and Kleinman, 2003; Fryers, Melzer and Jenkins, 2003) and in countries in the global north (Lund et al., 2010). The implication is that mental health workers, including some psychiatrists, should move outside the clinic to collaborate with others as workers in public health. But while studies certainly demonstrate social determinants, they are also inconclusive and contradictory about exactly which aspects of social disadvantage are important – bad experiences in childhood, financial stress, poor housing, bad education, insecure employment, social isolation, etc.; each is sometimes found to be significant, and sometimes not. They are also unclear about whether objective material conditions account for this gradient, or whether subjective responses to those material conditions are decisive – a point to which I will return. The WHO report does rise to the challenge of mechanisms, however, suggesting that the mechanism that translates these diverse forms of disadvantage to mental distress is 'stress', especially prolonged and unrelieved, or 'toxic' stress, and that the malign effects of 'stress' can be 'buffered' by various forms of social support; again, I will return to this.[5]

Fourth, if we accept that there are social, cultural, environmental determinants of mental distress, we can now use novel research methodologies to grasp these in more detail. We have cohort studies that take epigenetic data alongside biographical, social and mental health measures across the life course, and help us understand the later life consequences of early adversities.[6] We have geomapping, which can produce much more accurate spatialisations of the relations between mental ill health and a range of environmental exposures than were possible before. We have mental health apps, coupled with geomapping, which can trace an individual's experienced mental health state and link it to their precise location in a city, to whether their anxiety may be more intense in crowds and less so in spaces, to the mental health consequences of long commutes or hazardous workspaces and much more.[7] And, perhaps less well known, we have a growing body of research methodologies enabling us to explore the experience of mental distress from the perspective of actual or potential psychiatric service users: the rise of new methods and concepts from the service user's perspective challenges the 'monologue of reason over madness' and the authority of 'expert' knowledge which it embodies (Campbell and Rose, 2010; Rose, 2017).

Fifth, we have seen the emergence – or I should say the re-emergence – of 'mental ill health in the city' as a governmental domain: a range of arguments that point to the prevalence of mental distress in specific cities, draw attention to its personal, familial, social and economic consequences, and prioritise policy interventions to address it. There is a long history of urban biopolitics of mental disorder, from the eugenic policies in the United States (US), Canada and many other cities in the late nineteenth and early twentieth centuries, through the ecological biopolitics linked to the Chicago School, to the mental hygiene movements of the inter-war years. Today, high-profile urban mental health programmes such as ThriveNYC in New York, Thrive LDN in London, the 'Big Anxiety' in Sydney and many others also start from arguments that the rate of mental ill health in the city is a major challenge. But they believe that it is possible, indeed necessary, to use urban policy to make the city 'thrive' again. These programmes contain a recurrent mix of policies. Take the six principles of ThriveNYC:

- 'Change the culture' to enable New Yorkers to have an open conversation about mental health, training people in ways of responding to those in mental distress and shifting the focus of mental health towards public health.
- 'Act early', prioritising preventive intervention especially in families and schools, repeating the familiar argument that earlier is almost always better, and early intervention services are key.
- 'Close treatment gaps' by providing mental health care provisions locally in every community and thus improving access and impact,

although a lot of the specific actions concern homelessness and opioid addiction.
- 'Partner with communities', embracing the wisdom and strength of local communities, to create effective and culturally competent solutions, which seems to amount to trying to create pathways to specialist care for those with mental health needs.
- 'Use better data', by collecting reliable city-wide data on the health and emotional wellness of children and the factors affecting it, and establishing a mental health innovation laboratory to analyse and interpret the data.
- 'Strengthen government's ability to lead' by creating a mental health council to engage the community and implement the plans. The New York City Mental Health Commissioner Gary Belkin is passionately committed to making New York City a place where citizens can 'thrive', and this urban biopolitics of mental health certainly departs from its many predecessors in many ways, and is being emulated in a number of other cities, notably London and Toronto. But it is not clear that it draws upon social science research, or any of the 'biosocial' developments I have discussed here.

Nonetheless, in the confluence of these five dimensions, it seems to me that we are at an important point at which 'research and its results, despite their often intangible means, [might] make urban life visible through a different lens, [and] create concrete new urban experiences' in which research has a capacity to change the experience of urban life and urban mental distress.[8] Now as soon as one tries to incorporate social experiences and neurobiological mechanisms into a diagram to depict the relations between adversity and mental ill health, things get extremely complicated.[9] Faced with such complexity, which is probably the reality, it is no wonder that some yearn for the radical simplification of the laboratory experiment, despite the repeated evidence of the impossibility of translating the results from the protected and artificial space of the laboratory to the wild world outside (Callon, Lascoumes and Barthe, 2009). It is also no wonder that some take a different route and say: 'who cares about the detailed "causal architecture": we know at a population level that poverty, disadvantage, bad housing, insecure employment and the like are highly correlated with mental ill health, so why sweat over the details? When those major determinants have been mitigated, we can worry about how to deal with the pockets of mental distress that remain.' This view is undoubtedly appealing, and appears, in a more sophisticated form, in the arguments by Bruce Link and Jo Phelan about what they term 'fundamental causes' (Phelan and Link, 2013): research that tries to tease out the details of mechanisms, they say, often ignores what puts individuals 'at risk of risk'. 'Social factors such as socioeconomic status and social support are likely "fundamental causes" of disease that, because they embody access to important resources, affect multiple disease outcomes through multiple mechanisms, and consequently maintain an association with disease even when intervening mechanisms change' (Link and Phelan, 1995: 80).

But suppose we cared about mechanisms

Are mechanisms irrelevant once one finds correlations? No: mechanisms remain crucial. First, in the absence of an understanding of mechanisms we may think we can do nothing prior to a major transformation of our societies, since small changes leave fundamental causes untouched. Second, we may actually misidentify the roots of the problem and hence misdirect our interventions: consider, for example, the difference between interventions that result from the belief that mental disorders arise from multiple inherited genetic variations affecting the activity of neurotransmitters such as serotonin and dopamine, and those that might result from the belief that the mechanism is a stress-related disruption of the microbiome and the immune system, leading to increased susceptibility to chronic inflammation of the brain, as in some current research on schizophrenia and other serious disorders (Müller et al., 2015; Alam, Abdolmaleky and Zhou, 2017).[10]

The WHO report (2014) regarded adverse social conditions as causal, but studies are ambiguous about which dimensions of social disadvantage are key: education, food insecurity, housing, socio-economic status and financial stress exhibit a relatively consistent and strong association, while other simpler variables such as income and employment were more equivocal (Lund, 2014; Burns, 2015). The same is true of studies that have focused on the specific question of mental ill health in the urban environment, whether in relation to severe disorders such as schizophrenia (Krabbendam and Van Os, 2005) or on 'common mental disorders' such as depression and anxiety (Paykel et al., 2000; Gong et al., 2016; Fone et al., 2014).

Nonetheless the WHO report suggests a mechanism: 'stress'. Now the notion of stress has been used in everyday speech going back to the eighteenth century: stress as hardship, straits, adversity, affliction. In the nineteenth century many physical and emotional ills were blamed on the increasing stress of modern life (Jackson, 2013). By the end of the nineteenth century, the rapidly expanding cities were thought of as particularly stressful places. From the 1920s onwards, building on the work of Walter Cannon, researchers used animal models to understand the biology of stress, and Hans Selye announced his 'general adaptation syndrome': whatever the cause of stress in his rats – heat, cold, injections of noxious substances, etc. – the biological response was the same: stimulation of the adrenal glands to prepare the animal for 'fight or flight' (Selye, 1936). And when this stress response was prolonged in situations where the animal was unable to escape, this led to all manner of physical and behavioural pathologies.

This work was taken up in relation to overcrowding in the experiments of John Calhoun, examined by Ed Ramsden (Adams and Ramsden, 2011; Ramsden, 2011; Cantor and Ramsden, 2014; Ramsden, 2014).[11] Behavioural pathologies in overcrowded rat colonies led to the development of 'behavioural sinks', to use Calhoun's term, where female rats 'fell short of their maternal functions', infant mortality increased, and, for the males, 'behavior disturbances ranged from sexual deviation to cannibalism and from frenetic overactivity to a pathological withdrawal from which individuals would emerge to eat, drink and move about only when other members of the community were asleep. The social organisation of the animals showed equal disruption.'

For those involved in city planning in the US in the 1960s and 1970s, the stress responses to overcrowding in rats had obvious lessons for humans, and this generated a fierce debate about the effects of urban density. These questions were taken up by a large interdisciplinary group in the US containing many leading social scientists and urbanists, the Committee on Physical and Social Environmental Variables as Determinants of Mental Health, which met biannually from 1956 to 1968 (Duhl, 1963). The language of stress became a potent and highly transferrable framework for coding the challenges to human health in multiple domains – in the military, the factory, in everyday life in the modern world – and in the city. International conferences were held in the US and the United Kingdom (UK), extensive volumes were published linking stress to all manner of diseases of the body and of the mind (Kirk, 2014), and it seemed that almost all key figures – biologists, psychiatrists, psychologists, physiologists, ethnologists, sociologists, architects and planners – sought to think through the ways to link the physical and social spaces of the city to the mental health of citizens via the intermediary of stress.

These endeavours in the 1950s, 1960s and 1970s by and large came to a pretty depressing end. This was for three reasons. The first was that although most of the participants used the term 'stress', they meant very different things by it. Interdisciplinary conversations were achieved at the price of recognising and coming to terms with these differences. Secondly there was no agreement as to whether stress was something objective in the physical or social environment, or a subjective perception and experience, such that what was stressful for one person or one social or cultural or ethnic group, or women rather than men, or the old rather than the young, was not stressful to others. There was much research on 'stress' in urban environments: the stress of commuting, noise, crowding and much more. Amos Rapoport was probably speaking for most researchers on urban stress in humans when he concluded, in 1978, that stress was not 'objective' but depended on a subjective perception of particular environments and hence was shaped by culture, biography, language, symbols and meaning (Rapoport, 1978).[12] Thirdly, while most agreed that stress occurs when the organism's homeostatic mechanisms are unable to maintain a state of dynamic equilibrium, which impairs psychological functioning, it was by no means clear how such stress might lead to physical disease or mental disorder.

Many abandoned stress research for these reasons. But by the 1990s, stress came to the fore again, equipped with an updated neurobiological foundation. In their much cited paper of 1993, Bruce McEwen and Elliot Stellar argued that prolonged experience of stress in humans increased 'allostatic load' – the 'strain on the body produced by repeated ups and downs of physiologic response [to stress], as well as by the elevated activity of physiologic systems under challenge, and the changes in metabolism and the impact of wear and tear on a number of organs and tissues' and argued that prolonged increases in allostatic load led to 'specific changes in the immune and cardiovascular systems and neural and adipose tissues that produce specific disease outcomes' (McEwen and Stellar, 1993: 2094). Crucially, stress was now a mental and indeed cerebral phenomenon. As McEwen puts it in a paper entitled 'Brain on stress: How the social environment gets under the skin', the brain is 'the central organ of stress and adaptation': 'Stress is a state of the mind, involving both brain and body as well as their interactions' (McEwen, 2012: 17180).

The brain shapes what is perceived as stressful, and determines the consequences of that stress. The social and the physical environment gets 'under the skull' because of the way it is perceived and understood (Davidson and McEwen, 2012). In humans, McEwan argues, culturally shaped perceptions that one is in a stressful, pressured or threatening situation act on the structural plasticity of the hippocampus and other brain regions, notably the amygdala, the prefrontal cortex and the nucleus acumbens. A key mechanism for such changes is epigenetic – that is to say, via the regulation of gene expression. Animal studies show that both acute and chronic stress produces neuronal changes, inhibiting neurogenesis and affecting synaptic turnover, spine density, branching and length of neuronal axons; many of these studies have been supported by neuroimaging studies in humans. Repeated stress 'causes functional changes in neural circuitry in the hypothalamus' (Senst and Bains, 2014: 102), which alters activation of the immune system: continued activation of the immune system produces cytokines that act on other cells, leading to behaviour changes and depression-like symptoms (Dantzer et al., 2008; Pariante and Lightman, 2008) – popularly known as the 'inflamed brain' or 'inflamed mind' thesis.[13]

Many focus on the long-term effects of 'toxic' stress in childhood, which, McEwen argues, has 'implications for understanding health disparities and the impact of early life adversity and for intervention and prevention strategies' (McEwen, 2013: 673). Writing with his brother Craig, a sociologist, he makes the dubious claim that toxic stress in childhood can help account for the reproduction of poverty in families across generations in the US – dubious when many factors such as poor schooling, financial hardship and racial discrimination seem more obvious and proximal causes.

As Manning has pointed out (2019), the evidence that allostatic load is consistently linked to broad indices of social deprivation such as socio-economic status is equivocal, at least in part because of the heterogeneity of measures used (Dowd, Simanek and Aiello, 2009; Johnson, Cavallaro and Leon, 2017). Nonetheless, such research seems to identify one pathway for the corporeal and cerebral consequences of adversity. In a paper entitled 'Six paths for the future of social epidemiology', Sandro Galea and Bruce Link argued that if social epidemiology was to distinguish itself from other branches of epidemiology it had to address causes and mechanism (Galea and Link, 2013). As already mentioned, Link, with Jo Phelan, has long argued that socio-economic status is a 'fundamental social cause' (Link and Phelan, 1995; Phelan and Link, 2010), but Galea focused on the role of epigenetic changes that modify gene expression and activated molecular pathways to mental disorder. His group found distinctive gene methylation profiles in residents of a Detroit neighbourhood who had been assaulted, and suggested that 'cumulative traumatic burden may leave a molecular footprint in those with [PTSD]' (Galea, Uddin and Koenen, 2011: 402) and more generally that 'different aspects of the urban environment are distinctly and variably linked to brain structure, function, and hence phenotype' (Galea, 2011: 859). But some individuals and groups in incredibly 'stressful' circumstances seem to survive and thrive: why?

Buffering stress

The WHO report suggests that the link between social status and mental disorder may be shaped by 'the level, frequency and duration of stressful experiences and the extent to which they are buffered by social supports in the community' and that those 'lower on the social hierarchy' are more likely to be subject to such experiences, and have access to fewer buffers and supports (WHO, 2014: 16–18). This idea of 'buffering' by social supports draws upon the one seemingly sociological concept that regularly figures in neuropsychiatric research: 'social capital'. Many researchers argue that high 'social capital' is conducive to mental health because it is protective (Muntaner, 2004; Kelleher, 2003; Sartorius, 2003; Dannenberg et al., 2003; Saegert and Evans, 2003; McKenzie, Whitley and Weich, 2002; Henderson and Whiteford, 2003). This is not the place to trace the complex roots of this idea; in this literature on mental health it is a fuzzy concept, oscillating between attention to the material conditions of life – stable families, established communities, social integration, access to mental care and so forth – and a focus on what is termed 'cognitive social capital', that is to say an individual's *feelings* of trust and *beliefs* that he or she exists in a web of mutual obligations and reciprocality. Sadly, while it is initially appealing – for who would not believe that such social bonds were conductive to mental health and protective in times of adversity? – the evidence is inconclusive. But the results of empirical investigations are confused, not only because of the variety of ways in which this notion has been conceptualised, but by the diversity of ways it has been operationalised in attempts to measure it, and because of the naivety in thinking of social capital 'in isolation from the political and historical context of any given society' (Almedom, 2005: 946).

We can see the ambiguous consequences of such a focus on 'buffers' in the WHO report on social determinants. The report suggests that 'toxic stress' in childhood – strong and frequent or prolonged adversity such as abuse, neglect, violence and economic hardship, over a long period without adequate support – is 'buffered by social support provided by loving, responsive and stable relationships with a caring adult' (WHO, 2014: 18) which is less likely if mothers are young, socially or economically disadvantaged, experiencing a hostile or violent environment or themselves suffering from mental health problems. Schooling and home support throughout childhood, they suggest, can build 'emotional resilience', and this too is less likely for children in families living in poverty and stressful circumstances: hence they argue that efforts to support poorer families, especially those where adults themselves are suffering poor mental health will 'help disrupt the intergenerational transfer of inequities' (WHO, 2014: 27). Many would agree with their key message that 'Mental health and many common mental disorders are shaped to a great extent by the social, economic and physical environments in which people live.' But it is easy to interpret these arguments about the key role of mothers and families in childhood as a reprise of earlier views on 'the cycle of deprivation' (Joseph, 1972) rewritten in neural terms, views that led to policies directed at poor families themselves rather than at the social conditions that thrust them into poverty (Welshman, 2007).

Another biopolitics

Research on stress is of interest because it illustrates the long history of interactions between social scientists and life scientists. It is also interesting because it seems to have identified mechanisms by which a variety of subjective experiences, perceived as stressful as a result of individual biography, culturally shaped meanings and environmental insults, can be translated into neurobiological configurations with deleterious consequences for brain and body. But the research also raises conceptual questions of how we might develop a finer-grained, ethnographically informed analysis of the accumulation of urban situations that constitute stress and their spatial, temporal and sensorial characteristics. In psychiatric research, stress usually appears to be an individual phenomenon. But sociological and ethnographic investigations should map out the ways in which the experience of stress, and of poverty, exclusion, isolation, racism and violence, are shaped by cultural narratives and beliefs. They should also examine what there might be, within collective urban life, that mitigates against stress, whether that be the physical environment, mundane experiences in cafes and corner shops, informal friendships or forms of cooperative organisation. What kind of biopolitics might such a neurosocial and neurocultural understanding of urban existence enable?

As I argued at the start of this chapter, in the face of arguments about the prevalence of mental ill health in their own cities, urban policy makers have attempted to reverse this relationship, to make their city a place where individuals and communities can 'thrive'. So in these emerging programmes for healthy cities, are we seeing 'evidence-based' programmes and policies for mental health in urban settings?

Let me return to the Thrive programme. While there is much here to admire, it has to be said that it is remarkably evidence-light. Despite the wish to engage communities and build partnerships, most of the interventions are top-down and professional-driven. And rather than seeking to understand what it is in New York City, or in other cities, that drives people to mental ill health, the strategy starts from the existence of what are assumed to be mental disorders and emphasises the need for these to be recognised early, and for those with such disorders or at risk of them to have early access to professional mental health services in the name of prevention. Communities are important, but, for Thrive, they need to be trained by professionals: professionals collaborating with communities, training communities and so forth. Little attention is paid to the fact that in reality, the vast majority of care for people experiencing mental distress is, and will continue to be, provided informally, outside the professional sector. What we call primary care in health services is actually secondary care, coming into action only for those selected few who – by processes well studied by sociologists and anthropologists – come to the attention of medical or other authorities (Porter, 1985). And, to the extent that we can draw anything from the research on social capital and social exclusion, these local informal networks are often threatened, professionalised or demoralised by the incursion of professionals.

The kinds of research I have discussed here suggest other strategies to address the social determinants of mental distress in urban settings. The path to mitigating mental ill health, and to maximising mental wellbeing, does not lie through the mental health services or allied professionals as currently conceived: it lies in directly addressing those determinants in the light of more precise knowledge of the mechanisms through which they act, and by which they can be mitigated. It lies in understanding the capabilities that are required to lead a fulfilled life, and the resources necessary to realise these capabilities (Nussbaum, 2011). This may well require a complete reconstruction of mental health services, a retraining of professionals and greatly enhanced powers for those who have experienced mental distress and who understand mental health services from the point of view of those who have been their subjects – not an easy task but a necessary one if one is to learn the lessons from social research (Rose, 2018).

In conclusion

The Urban Brain programme is an experiment to see if it is possible to conduct such neurosocial and neurocultural research into specific and urgent socio-political questions. As I have said, it focuses on rural–urban migration in Shanghai and São Paulo, with comparators in the different migrant cities of Toronto and London. The research analyses epidemiological, psychiatric and ethnographic data, including our own research on mental health of migrants, to draw a thick picture of migrant life at work, at home and on the street. It uses conventional instruments to evaluate the mental health of a sample of the migrant population in different types of work and different forms of dwelling. It uses a range of measures to assess 'stress'. It involves partnership with psychiatrists, architects, artists and urban geographers to construct an 'urban mind' smartphone app to track mood across time and space, sampling both the physical environment and the urban sensorium. And it entails collaboration with other researchers working on the exposome and the microbiome, to obtain measures of the 'atmosphere' of the migrant city.

The research asks whether it is possible to rework Margaret Lock's idea of local biologies in ecological terms (Lock and Kaufert, 2001). While urban ecology is much derided these days, perhaps it could be helpful to think of the urban experience in terms of an array of niches, or habitats, what we term biological localities. The idea of a 'biological locality' helps us to rethink the dynamics and rhythms of urban spaces, as they make and remake exchanges of wealth and poverty, of power and exclusion, of exposures and atmospheres, of surveillance and security, of mobility and stasis, worry, anxiety, uncertainty and precarity, of community and isolation. In seeking to integrate biological and neurobiological insights and methods with older questions about inequality, poverty, exclusion, racism and violence, this research hopes to contribute to an urban biopolitics that does not focus on the diagnosis and therapeutics of the pathological individual, but addresses the pathogenic features of urban forms of life themselves. What might it mean to imagine 'the good city' through a neurosocial lens? Could we redeploy the language of biopolitics not for critique of metropolitan governments, but as a way to rethink the politics of health, stress and exposure in cities? If the urban experience is instantiated neurobiologically, a *positive* biopolitics of urban space would require us to think normatively, to ask whether a neurosocial style of thought might help us to clarify what we might hope for in shaping a good life, a flourishing life in the contemporary city.

Acknowledgements

This chapter draws on many discussions in the Neuroscience and Society Research Network and with my colleagues in the Urban Brain Project, including two recent papers written with Des Fitzgerald and Ilina Singh (Fitzgerald, Rose and Singh, 2016a; Fitzgerald, Rose and Singh, 2016b). It also draws on ongoing discussions with Nick Manning on questions of mechanisms (for more details see Manning, 2019). In addition to this, the chapter draws on research supported by the following grants: the European Union's Horizon 2020 Research and Innovation Programme funding for the *Human Brain Project* under Grant Agreement No. 720270; ESRC Award ES/L003074/1: *A New Sociology for a New Century: Transforming the Relations between Sociology and Neuroscience, through a Study of Mental Life*; ESRC-NSFC Award ES/N010892/1: *Urban Transformations in China*; and an award for *Mental Health, Migration and the Mega City (Sao Paulo) – M3SP* from King's-FAPESP APR Scheme.

Notes

1 See WHO, www.who.int/sustainable-development/cities/Factsheet-Cities-sustainable-health.pdf?ua=1 (last accessed 1 November 2019).
2 For more information about the Urban Brain Programme, see https://urbanbrainlab.com/ (last accessed 15 October 2019). This is also the topic

of the book that I am writing with Des Fitzgerald called *The Urban Brain: Mental health in the vital city*, to be published by Princeton University Press in 2020.
3 For more information about South East London Community Health, see www.kcl.ac.uk/ioppn/depts/pm/research/selcoh/about/index.aspx (last accessed 15 October 2019).
4 With acknowledgements to the late Ian Dury: www.youtube.com/watch?v=qcjh1a9Yoao (last accessed 15 October 2019).
5 For a quick introduction to contemporary beliefs about stress and toxic stress, see https://developingchild.harvard.edu/science/key-concepts/toxic-stress/ (last accessed 15 October 2019).
6 Such as the ALSPAC study: www.bristol.ac.uk/alspac/ (last accessed 15 October 2019).
7 For example, the Urban Mind App, which we are helping develop in collaborator with Andrea Mechelli and his group at King's College London: www.urbanmind.info/ (last accessed 15 October 2019).
8 This was part of the rationale for the workshop in Rio de Janeiro at which a draft of this chapter was first presented.
9 See, for example, the figures illustrating stress pathways in McEwen and Stellar's classic paper in McEwen and Stellar, 1993, or Pescolido's diagram of the NEM III R (Network Episode Model) in Pescosolido, 2011.
10 My colleague Nick Manning points to the implications of the long-held belief that stomach ulcers arose from personality and lifestyle, rather than infection with Helicobacter pylori.
11 The following paragraphs are indebted to Ramsden's work, which he presented at our first Urban Brain workshop in 2013.
12 A tiny example: in our current research in Shanghai, a young women migrant from Shandong, in discussion with our resident ethnographer, Lisa Richaud, said how much she enjoyed travelling on the unbelievably crowded Shanghai metro in the rush hours, it gave her a feeling of collective momentum (*dongli*) and she liked feeling part of that.
13 'The Inflamed Mind' was the title of a BBC documentary in August 2016, available at www.bbc.co.uk/programmes/b07pj2pw (last accessed 15 October 2019).

References

Adams, J. and Ramsden, E. (2011). Rat cities and beehive worlds: Density and design in the modern city. *Comparative Studies in Society and History*, 53(4): 722–56.

Alam, R., Abdolmaleky, H.M., and Zhou, J. R. (2017). Microbiome, inflammation, epigenetic alterations, and mental diseases. *American Journal of Medical Genetics Part B: Neuropsychiatric Genetics*, 174(6): 651–60.

Almedom, A.M. (2005). Social capital and mental health: An interdisciplinary review of primary evidence. *Social Science & Medicine*, 61(5): 943–64.

Benton, T. (1993) *Natural relations: Ecology, animal rights and social justice*. London: Verso.

Bhugra, D., Tasman, A., Pathare, S., Priebe, S., Smith, S., Torous, J., Arbuckle, M.R., Langford, A., Alarcón, R.D., and Chiu, H.F.K. (2017). The WPA–Lancet Psychiatry Commission on the future of psychiatry. *Lancet Psychiatry*, 4(10): 775–818.

Burns, J. (2015). Poverty, inequality and a political economy of mental health. *Epidemiology and Psychiatric Sciences*, 24(02): 107–13.

Callon, M., Lascoumes, P., and Barthe, Y. (2009). *Acting in an uncertain world: An essay on technical democracy*. Cambridge, MA: MIT Press.

Campbell, P., and Rose, D. (2010). Action for change in the UK: Thirty years of the user/survivor movement. In D. Pilgrim, A. Rogers and B. Pescosolido (eds), *The SAGE handbook of mental health and illness*, 452–70. Newcastle: Sage.

Campion, J., Bhugra, D., Bailey, S., and Marmot, M. (2013). Inequality and mental disorders: Opportunities for action. *Lancet*, 382(9888): 183–4.

Cantor, D. and Ramsden, E. (2014). *Stress, shock, and adaptation in the twentieth century*. Rochester, NY: University of Rochester Press.

Dannenberg, A.L., Jackson, R.J., Frumkin, H., Schieber, R.A., Pratt, M., Kochtitzky, C., and Tilson, H.H. (2003). The impact of community design and land-use choices on public health: A scientific research agenda. *American Journal of Public Health*, 93(9): 1500–8.

Dantzer, R., O'Connor, J.C., Freund, G.G., Johnson, R.W., and Kelley, K.W. (2008). From inflammation to sickness and depression: When the immune system subjugates the brain. *Nature Reviews Neuroscience*, 9(1): 46–56.

Davidson, R.J., and McEwen, B.S. (2012). Social influences on neuroplasticity: Stress and interventions to promote well-being. *Nature Neuroscience*, 15(5): 689–95.

Dowd, J.B., Simanek, A.M., and Aiello, A.E. (2009). Socio-economic status, cortisol and allostatic load: A review of the literature. *International Journal of Epidemiology*, 38(5): 1297–1309.

Duhl, L. (1963). *The urban condition: People and policy in the metropolis*. New York: Basic Books.

Fassin, D. (2009). Another politics of life is possible. *Theory, Culture & Society*, 26(5): 44–60.

Fitzgerald, D., Rose, N., and Singh, I. (2016a). Living well in the neuropolis. *The Sociological Review Monographs*, 64(1): 221–37.

Fitzgerald, D., Rose, N., and Singh, I. (2016b). Revitalizing sociology: Urban life and mental illness between history and the present. *The British Journal of Sociology*, 67(1): 138–60.

Fone, D., White, J., Farewell, D., Kelly, M., John, G., Lloyd, K., Williams, G., and Dunstan, F. (2014). Effect of neighbourhood deprivation and social cohesion on mental health inequality: A multilevel population-based longitudinal study. *Psychological Medicine*, 44(11): 2449–60.

Fryers, T., Melzer, D., and Jenkins, R. (2003). Social inequalities and the common mental disorders. *Social Psychiatry and Psychiatric Epidemiology*, 38(5): 229–37.

Galea, S. (2011). The urban brain: New directions in research exploring the relation between cities and mood–anxiety disorders. *Depression and Anxiety*, 28: 857–62.

Galea, S., and Link, B.G. (2013). Six paths for the future of social epidemiology. *American Journal of Epidemiology*, 178(6): 843–49.

Galea, S., Uddin, M., and Koenen, K. (2011). The urban environment and mental disorders: Epigenetic links. *Epigenetics*, 6(4): 400–4.

Gong, Y., Palmer, S., Gallacher, J., Marsden, T., and Fone, D. (2016). A systematic review of the relationship between objective measurements of the urban environment and psychological distress. *Environment International*, 96: 48–57.

Grosz, E.A. (1994). *Volatile bodies: Toward a corporeal feminism*. Bloomington and Indianapolis: Indiana University Press.

Henderson, S., and Whiteford, H. (2003). Social capital and mental health. *Lancet*, 362(9383): 505–6.

Jackson, M. (2013). *The age of stress: Science and the search for stability*. Oxford: Oxford University Press.

Johnson, S.C., Cavallaro, F.L., and Leon, D.A. (2017). A systematic review of allostatic load in relation to socioeconomic position: Poor fidelity and major inconsistencies in biomarkers employed. *Social Science & Medicine*, 192: 66–73.

Joseph, K. (1972). The cycle of deprivation. *Midwife and Health Visitor*, 8(12): 414.

Kelleher, C. (2003). Mental health and 'the Troubles' in Northern Ireland: Implications of civil unrest for health and wellbeing. *Journal of Epidemiology and Community Health*, 57: 474–5.

Kirk, R.G.W. (2014). The invention of the 'stressed animal' and the development of a science of animal welfare, 1947–86. In D. Cantor and E. Ramsden (eds), *Stress, shock, and adaptation in the twentieth century*, 241–63. Rochester, NY: University of Rochester Press.

Krabbendam, L., and Van Os, J. (2005). Schizophrenia and urbanicity: A major environmental influence – conditional on genetic risk. *Schizophrenia Bulletin*, 31(4): 795–9.

Link, B.G., and Phelan, J. (1995). Social conditions as fundamental causes of disease. *Journal of Health and Social Behavior*, extra issue: *Forty years of medical sociology: The state of the art and directions for the future*, 80–94.

Lock, M., and Kaufert, P. (2001). Menopause, local biologies, and cultures of aging. *American Journal of Human Biology*, 13(4): 494–504.

Lund, C. (2014). Poverty and mental health: Towards a research agenda for low and middle-income countries. *Social Science & Medicine*, 111: 134–6.

Lund, C., Breen, A., Flisher, A. J., Kakuma, R., Corrigall, J., Joska, J.A., Swartz, L., and Patel, V. (2010). Poverty and common mental disorders in low and middle income countries: A systematic review. *Social Science & Medicine*, 71(3): 517–28.

Manning, N. (2019). Sociology, biology and mechanisms in urban mental health. *Social Theory and Health*, 17(10): 1–22.

McEwen, B. S. (2012). Brain on stress: How the social environment gets under the skin. *Proceedings of the National Academy of Sciences*, 109 (supplement 2): 17180–5.

McEwen, B.S. (2013). The brain on stress: Toward an integrative approach to brain, body, and behavior. *Perspectives on Psychological Science*, 8(6): 673–5.

McEwen, B.S., and Stellar, E. (1993). Stress and the individual: Mechanisms leading to disease. *Archives of Internal Medicine*, 153(18): 2093–2101.

McKenzie, K., Whitley, R., and Weich, S. (2002). Social capital and mental health. *British Journal of Psychiatry*, 181(4): 280–3.

Meloni, M., Williams, S., and Martin, P. (2016). The biosocial: Sociological themes and issues. *The Sociological Review Monographs*, 64(1): 7–25.

Müller, N., Weidinger, E., Leitner, B., and Schwarz, M.J. (2015). The role of inflammation in schizophrenia. *Frontiers in Neuroscience*, 9: 372.

Muntaner, C. (2004). Commentary: Social capital, social class, and the slow progress of psychosocial epidemiology. *International Journal of Epidemiology*, 33(4): 674–80.

Nussbaum, M. C. (2011). *Creating capabilities*. Cambridge, MA: Harvard University Press.

Pariante, C.M. and Lightman, S.L. (2008). The HPA axis in major depression: Classical theories and new developments. *Trends in Neurosciences*, 31(9): 464–8.

Patel, V. and Kleinman, A. (2003). Poverty and common mental disorders in developing countries. *Bulletin of the World Health Organization*, 81(8): 609–15.

Patel, V., Lund, C., Hatherill, S., Plagerson, S., Corrigall, J., Funk, M., and Flisher, A. (2010). Mental disorders: Equity and social determinants. In E. Blas and A.S. Kurup (eds), *Equity, social determinants and public health programmes*, 115–34. Geneva: WHO.

Paykel, E., Abbott, R., Jenkins, R., Brugha, T., and Meltzer, H. (2000). Urban-rural mental health differences in Great Britain: Findings from the National Morbidity Survey. *Psychological Medicine*, 30(2): 269–80.

Pescosolido, B.A. (2011). Organizing the sociological landscape for the next decades of health and health care research: The network episode model Iii-R as cartographic subfield guide. In B.A. Pescosolido, J.K. Martin, J.D. McLeod and A. Rogers, *Handbook of the sociology of health, illness, and healing*, 39–66. New York: Springer.

Phelan, J.C., and Link, B.G. (2010). Fundamental social causes of health inequalities. In C. Morgan and D. Bhugra (eds), *Principles of social psychiatry*, 181–92. Chichester: Wiley.

Phelan, J. C. and Link, B. G. (2013). Fundamental cause theory. In W.C. Cockerham (ed.). *Medical sociology on the move*, 105–25. London: Springer.

Porter, R. (1985). The patient's view. *Theory and Society*, 14(2): 175–98.

Ramsden, E. (2011). From rodent utopia to urban hell: Population, pathology, and the crowded rats of Nimh. *Isis*, 102(4): 659–88.

Ramsden, E. (2014). Stress in the city: Mental health, urban planning and the social sciences in the postwar United States. In D. Cantor and E. Ramsden (eds), *Stress, shock and adaptation in the twentieth century*, 291–319. Rochester, NY: University of Rochester Press.

Rapoport, A. (1978). Culture and the subjective effects of stress. *Urban Ecology*, 3(3): 241–61.

Rose, D. (2017). Service user/survivor-led research in mental health: Epistemological possibilities. *Disability & Society*, 32(6): 1–17.

Rose, N. (2018). Our psychiatric future: The politics of mental health. Cambridge: Polity.

Rose, N., and Abi-Rached, J. M. (2013). *Neuro: The new brain sciences and the management of the mind*. Woodstock: Princeton University Press.

Rose, N., and Abi-Rached, J. M. (2014). Governing through the brain: Neuropolitics, neuroscience and subjectivity. *Cambridge Anthropology*, 32(1): 3–23.

Saegert, S., and Evans, G.W. (2003). Poverty, housing niches, and health in the United States. *Journal of Social Issues*, 59(3): 569–89.

Sartorius, N. (2003). Social capital and mental health. *Current Opinion in Psychiatry*, 16, S101–S105.

Selye, H. (1936). A syndrome produced by diverse nocuous agents. *Nature*, 138(3479): 32.

Senst, L., and Bains, J. (2014). Neuromodulators, stress and plasticity: A role for endocannabinoid signalling. *The Journal of Experimental Biology*, 217(1): 102–8.

Welshman, J. (2007). *From transmitted deprivation to social exclusion: Policy, poverty and parenting*. Bristol: Policy Press.

WHO (2014). Social Determinants of Mental Health. Geneva: WHO.

Wilson, E. A. (2015). *Gut feminism*. Durham, NC: Duke University Press.

# 3

Feminised urban futures, healthy cities and violence against women and girls: transnational reflections from Brazilians in London and Maré, Rio de Janeiro

Cathy McIlwaine, Miriam Krenzinger, Yara Evans and Eliana Sousa Silva

As women comprise a majority of urban citizens in the world today, questions remain about the nature of a feminised urban future. While it is established that urbanisation has the potential to promote gender transformations (Chant and McIlwaine, 2016), it is important to consider how positive changes are potentially undermined by violence against women and girls (VAWG) and, concomitantly, how violence affects women's health and wellbeing in cities. In a context whereby one in three women globally experiences such violence, with arguably higher incidence in cities (McIlwaine, 2013; UN Women, 2015), there is therefore an urgent need to explore these relationships. This chapter examines these issues in relation to wider debates on the gender-blindness of right to the city discourse and the importance of considering gender justice and wellbeing in cities (Moser, 2016), as well as the need to acknowledge cities as globally connected urban systems underpinned by gendered power relations (Peake and Reiker, 2013). The discussion draws empirically on the transnational nature of urban VAWG among Brazilian migrant women in London and those residing in the marginalised slums of one of Rio de Janeiro's largest favelas, Complexo da Maré. It shows how gender-based violence (GBV) is diverse across multiple spaces of the city in both contexts and how it fundamentally undermines women's wellbeing. Yet, while GBV emerges as a major barrier to ensuring equitable and healthy feminised urban futures, such futures are paradoxical. Although the roots of gendered violence lie in patriarchal power relations, it is exacerbated by other forms of indirect structural violence that relate to the challenges of living in cities in the global north and south at local and geopolitical scales (Pain, 2014; Philo, 2017). Yet urban living can also lead to improvements in women's lives, not least through better provision of support systems and services for women survivors of violence in comparison to those in rural areas.

Conceptualising feminised and healthy urban futures: The centrality of VAWG

Although urbanisation processes have long been acknowledged as gendered in terms of women and men experiencing cities differently (Chant, 2013), the treatment of gender in understanding cities has been more variegated. Indeed, discourses on the meaning of 'just' cities tend to neglect the gendered nature of urban justice (Moser, 2016). In turn, urban theorising has arguably been masculinist in nature (Peake, 2016) with feminist analyses of Lefebvrian formulation of urban rights being widely recognised as gender blind (Vacchelli and Kofman, 2018). Central to these debates has been the acknowledgement that women's experiences in the city cannot be divorced from the private sphere (Fenster, 2005), nor from the intersections between the private and the public (Peake, 2017). It is only in exploring the gendered links between the private and public spheres in the city that a more comprehensive understanding of GBV can be established (Datta, 2016). Women's right to the city therefore revolves not only around the absence of violence and fear, but also the importance of women's rights to ensure their good health and wellbeing as well as gender equality across all domains (Whitzman, Andrew and Viswanath, 2014).

Understanding VAWG more fully is therefore a key element in the debates around the contradictory nature of urban gender transformations in light of the fact that cities render wider configurations of gender norms and practices visible (Bondi and Christie, 2003). Cities can offer women scope to escape some domestic labour demands, access better remunerated paid work and potentially lead to shifts towards independence and self-development (Bradshaw, 2013; Hindin and Adair, 2002). Yet cities and urbanisation also create new demands for women in terms of providing new types of exploitative employment, creating time poverty, and the existence of urban problems in terms of air pollution and mobility challenges and so on (Chant and McIlwaine, 2016; McIlwaine, 2013), all of which undermine their health and wellbeing (DeVerteuil, 2015). As such, the notion of the city as liberating for women needs to be tempered (Peake, 2017), especially the 'healthy city', in light of the ways in which VAWG acts as a barrier to allowing women to fulfil their rights and wellbeing (UN Women, 2015).

Although GBV has often been marginalised as an issue in many cities, especially in those with very high levels of male homicide rates (Wilding, 2010; Wilding, 2012) or political violence (Esser, 2014), it is nonetheless endemic throughout the urban world. Although the relationship between GBV and urbanisation is not uniform, there is a growing consensus that women experience especially high levels of insecurity and violence in cities (Moser and McIlwaine, 2014). The most broadly accepted definitions of VAWG refer to violence where women and girls are targeted specifically because of their gender (Watts and Zimmermann, 2002) and the reasons for such violence are rooted in the exercise of social, economic or political power on the part of men against women, entailing the use of physical, sexual and psychological force and/or control in private and public spheres (McIlwaine, 2013). Acknowledging constraints of accurate data collection, evidence shows that non-intimate partner violence (non-IPV) in cities is higher than in rural areas, whereas intimate partner violence (IPV) is lower (McIlwaine, 2013). While globally, an estimated 35 per cent of women have experienced some form of GBV (World Health Organization (WHO), 2013: 12), UN-Habitat (2006) suggests that they are twice as likely to experience violence in cities, especially in the global south. Yet the nature of VAWG in cities everywhere is hugely diverse, and the incidence is higher in some parts and spaces of cities such as in slum communities of the south (Chant and McIlwaine, 2016). Although the root causes of VAWG lie in unequal gendered power relations, there are a host of urban conditions or forms of structural violence that can create 'stress-inducing conditions' that make gendered violence more likely to occur (Hindin and Adair, 2002). Poor-quality housing where residence is insecure, overcrowded and/or in makeshift dwellings can make women vulnerable to burglary, theft and multiple forms of sexual violence (Chant, 2013), together with lack of street lighting and restricted access to safe and affordable transport (McIlwaine, 2016). In turn, in slum communities where sanitary facilities are located far from people's homes it has emerged that women experience heightened levels of GBV, especially at night (Bapat and Agarwal, 2003). Urban public spaces can be sites of risk for women linked not only with lack of infrastructure, but also with the proliferation of places where drugs and alcohol are sold and consumed, contributing to increased levels of street-based gendered violence (Moser and McIlwaine, 2004). Urban poverty can also intersect with GBV, itself closely interrelated with lack of asset ownership, which can also make it more difficult for women to exit violent relationships (WHO, 2002).

These urban conditions rooted in various forms of structural and systemic violence also intersect with the health dimensions of urban VAWG (DeVerteuil, 2015). Indeed, it is worth pointing out that much early work on understanding VAWG was situated within a public health approach that framed it as a disease. For instance, Lori Heise's (1998) integrated ecological model for theorising the etiology of GBV identified a series of multidimensional interrelations between individual, situational and sociocultural factors as causal layers all underpinned by unequal gendered power relations. The ecological model is now recognised as the key theoretical foundation for research and programme work (Michau et al., 2015), especially by international agencies such as the WHO (2002) as well as in relation to understanding urban violence (Moser and McIlwaine, 2004). A key aspect of the public health approach is recognition of the multiple physiological and psychological effects of gendered violence, which include fractures and haemorrhaging, miscarriage, stillbirth, anxiety and post-traumatic stress disorder (PTSD) as well as greater susceptibility to human immunodeficiency virus (HIV) and sexually transmitted infections (STIs) (WHO, 2013: 21–2). These intersect with harmful alcohol and drug consumption, depression and suicide, and rape-trauma syndrome. In turn, these undermine women's ability to participate fully in city life, both productively, in terms of loss of income due to ill health caused by GBV, and socially, where women survivors may withdraw from friendship and social networks because of shame, stigma or rejection (Heise, Ellsberg and Gottmoeller, 2002). Arguably these social costs affect families and children when female care-givers withdraw from this role, with subsequent negative intergenerational effects among children who witness VAWG (McIlwaine, 2016). These processes are also experienced in intersectional ways, with certain women more likely to experience violence than others according to their class, ethnic, racial and sexual identities, disability and so on. Of particular importance here is racial/ethnic minority and immigration status, with migrant and/or minority women residing in cities often experiencing heightened levels of GBV linked with the wider experiences of vulnerability and structural violence (Dominguez and Menjívar, 2014).

However, the paradox of experiences of urban VAWG is that cities can also provide refuge for women who experience GBV. In a context whereby patriarchal strictures can be more flexible in urban areas than in the countryside (Chant, 2013), tolerance of gendered violence tends to be lower in cities (Hindin and Adair, 2002), with women survivors more likely to seek and secure support (Heise, Ellsberg and Gottmoeller, 2002). Tolerance also varies according to country, being influenced by variations in criminal justice systems and prevailing attitudes towards violence as well as state and civil society resources available to devote to support services (Vacchelli, Kathrecha and Gyte, 2015). Where the city has replaced the nation as the main scale of intervention in relation to justice issues (Peake, 2017), it is essential to recognise that the nature of and responses to VAWG vary according to city, within a wider context of it fundamentally undermining gender justice everywhere.

Whatever the specifics of VAWG, it is has been recognised in international policy domains as a major issue since the 1990s (Moser and McIlwaine, 2014). Indeed, Sustainable Development Goal (SDG) 5 explicitly targets the elimination of 'all forms of violence against all women and girls in public and private spheres, including trafficking and sexual and other types of exploitation' and identifies eliminating GBV as a priority. SDG 11 on urbanisation recognises that women are generally more marginalised than men in cities, especially in relation to safe, inclusive and accessible, green and public spaces. Similarly, the UN-Habitat New Urban Agenda (NUA), launched in 2016, echoed a commitment to gender equality in cities, even if the final versions of it ended up marginalising women and girls as a special-interest and vulnerable group (Moser, 2017: 233–4). Yet the importance of addressing women's safety in cities has a long history, dating back as far as the 1980s in London, and to the 1990s in relation to women's safety audits especially but not exclusively linked to the UN-Habitat Safer Cities programme (Whitzman, Andrew and Viswanath, 2014). While criticisms of such approaches revolve around the focus on GBV in the public sphere and on symptoms over causes, there have been recent moves towards more holistic, feminist approaches that foreground women's rights to experience the city equitably (Tankel, 2011). The chapter now turns to explore these issues in relation to the nature of VAWG among Brazilians residing in London and among women living in the favela of Complexo da Maré in Rio de Janeiro, Brazil.

Urban VAWG in London and Rio de Janeiro: background and methodological framework

Exploring the ways in which VAWG is experienced among two relatively marginalised populations of women in two major cities of the world can shed important light on gender relations and the ways in which GBV serves as a barrier to women's full participation in city life. This section draws on research conducted between 2016 and 2018 in London with Brazilian migrants and in Rio de Janeiro with favela residents from the Complexo da Maré. The research in London was carried out in the context of a Brazilian population that is relatively new to the city, with most arriving since 2000 (McIlwaine and Bunge, 2016). Although estimates vary, the 2011 United Kingdom (UK) census reported 52,000 Brazilians nationally, with 61 per cent concentrated in London (Evans et al., 2015). While Brazilians tend to be well educated, many are concentrated in manual jobs, with up to a third having insecure immigration status (Evans et al., 2011). This can lead to high levels of marginalisation exacerbated by difficulties in speaking English (McIlwaine and Evans, 2018). While there are no estimates for the incidence of VAWG among the Brazilian population, in the UK in general in 2013, 1.2 million women experienced domestic abuse, 60,000 were raped, and two women a week were killed by a current or former partner (Rights of Women, 2013). It is also widely accepted that levels are higher among black and minority-ethnic (BME) and migrant women, with qualitative research among Latin Americans in London suggesting that one woman in four experiences VAWG (McIlwaine and Carlisle, 2011).

In terms of the research framework, twelve interviews with organisations providing assistance for migrants were carried out (Evans and McIlwaine, 2017). In addition, an online survey was carried out of 175 Brazilian women from all over London, which addressed whether GBV had been experienced in the UK and/or Brazil and, if so, the various forms it took. Although there were limitations to this approach, especially in terms of biasing respondents to those who were more educated and computer-literate, it allowed women to complete it anonymously. Indeed, those who completed it tended to be relatively young (74 per cent aged under fifty), well educated (72 per cent with university education), employed in professional and managerial jobs (53 per cent) and ethnically white (73 per cent). Most were from São Paulo (42 per cent), with 10 per cent from Rio de Janeiro, and 9 per cent each from Minas Gerais and Paraná. In turn, 69 per cent of women were married or in stable relationships, 15 per cent were separated or divorced, and 13 per cent were single, with just over half having children (55 per cent). While this profile reflects more privilege than has been reported in other research (Evans et al., 2015), in-depth interviews allowed for exploration of women's experiences with more precarious occupational and immigration status. In total, twenty-five in-depth interviews were conducted, twenty with women survivors who had been supported by the Latin American Women's Rights Service (LAWRS), our partner organisation, and five with women who were recruited randomly through Brazilian networks and who had not necessarily experienced GBV. Six focus groups were also carried out, five with women and one with men (a total of sixteen people), using various forms of participatory appraisal methods to explore the nature of VAWG. All the interviews and focus groups were conducted at the migrant organisation with a trained counsellor on hand in case their support was required.

In Rio de Janeiro, the research was conducted in Complexo da Maré, which is in the north of the city and comprises nearly four square kilometres and includes sixteen slums, making it one of the largest favelas. By 2013 it had a population of almost 140,000, of whom 51 per cent were women. Maré is generally characterised by high levels of poverty, inequality and public insecurity. Many residents have low (although increasing) levels of education and work in informal or self-employment. More than half identify as mixed-race, a third as white and less than 10 per cent as black. While many informal workers are street vendors or domestic workers, there is also a vibrant entrepreneurial culture with around 2,500 small businesses. Yet Maré is dominated by four of Rio de Janeiro's Armed Criminal Groups (ACGs): Comando Vermelho (CV – Red Command), Terceiro Comando (TC – Third Command), Amigos dos Amigos (ADA – Friends of Friends) and the Militia (current and ex-police officers operating as an armed criminal group) (Silva Sousa, 2017). It has also been the site of continual police operations: in 2017 there were forty-one police operations which resulted in forty-two deaths, forty-one people wounded and the closure of health posts and schools for forty-five and thirty-five days respectively (Krenzinger et al., 2018). In terms of VAWG, it has been estimated that 35 per cent of women nationally have suffered GBV, of which 80 per cent was perpetrated by a current or former partner (Guimarães and Pedroza, 2015; see also Kiss et al., 2012). In Rio de Janeiro in 2016, 396 women were victims of homicide, with one woman murdered every day (Krenzinger et al., 2018).

A similar methodological framework was mobilised in Maré. This entailed mapping of fourteen service providers that address VAWG, together with a face-to-face questionnaire survey of 801 women together with seven focus groups with older women, female members of local religious organisations, LGBTQ+ people, drug users, community activists (male and female) and the field researchers (fifty-nine people in total across all groups). The fieldwork was carried out by researchers via Redes da Maré (our partner organisation) in three areas covering fifteen favelas using sequential sampling based on a prior census of the area. The survey had limitations relating to women's inhibitions in speaking freely about violence, due to the constant presence of members of armed groups. The survey showed that the women were predominantly young (65 per cent aged under forty-four), with the majority (62 per cent) born in Rio de Janeiro, of whom 41 per cent were born in Maré. Most women had limited education (53 per cent had only primary schooling); almost half identified as mixed-ethnicity (48 per cent) and 30 per cent stated they were white. In turn, 23 per cent of the women were in employment, and 21 per cent unemployed; another fifth worked on their own account, usually a small business. The remainder identified as home makers (19 per cent), retired (12 per cent) or students (2 per cent). More than a third (36 per cent) were single, 45 per cent married or in a stable relationship and 10 per cent separated or divorced, with 80 per cent having children.

The contexts of the two research sites, while fundamentally different in many ways, also share similarities in that women reside in various forms of marginal spaces of the city. Women in London face major challenges of insecurity in relation to their livelihoods, legal status and language competence, and in Maré they confront difficulties in relation to livelihoods, endemic urban violence and precarity. These challenges affect women's experiences of the city in ways that are exacerbated by GBV, to which the chapter now turns.

Multidimensionality of urban VAWG in London and Rio de Janeiro

The nature of VAWG emerged as multidimensional and multi-sited across private and public spheres by multiple perpetrators and over time. This multidimensionality can be viewed as a continuum whereby diverse types of physical and non-physical GBV intersect across scales from the individual to families, communities, cities and states, and transnationally (McIlwaine and Evans, 2020). Many women in London and Maré acknowledged that they were not aware of what VAWG constituted, especially non-physical violence among conjugal partners. For example, in London, forty-two-year-old Marcia was unaware until she visited a migrant organisation:

> All these years, 22 years, I didn't think I was suffering domestic violence, with the exception of the time when he punched me. But when I read the information on the leaflet, I was shocked to find that I had spent half my life suffering psychological, emotional abuse, without realising it.

Similarly, in Maré, a community leader from a focus group noted:

> When violence is psychological the woman takes much longer to understand that it is violence. Words also hurt, mistreat. There are women who have low self-esteem because they hear a lot of things they don't like and they get overwhelmed and sad.

Indeed, the Maré survey gave women the opportunity to define GBV for themselves, and it is notable that most associated it with physical aggression (56 per cent) while 10 per cent were unable to define it, which is potentially indicative of its ubiquity.

In terms of the incidence of VAWG, in London, where awareness was higher, 82 per cent of women reported having experienced it. Those most likely to report it had lived in the city for between ten and twenty years, were in their forties, educated to postgraduate level and of mixed race rather than white, were separated or divorced, worked in services and had access to their own income. As for the broad types identified, the most common was psychological/emotional violence (48 per cent), followed by physical violence (38 per cent) and sexual violence (14 per cent). Unwelcome physical contact was the commonest specific form of GBV (experienced by 42 per cent), together with physical assault (36 per cent) and being humiliated or suffering discrimination (33 per cent). The majority of perpetrators were known to women (66 per cent); although one third of GBV was committed by strangers, almost a quarter (23 per cent) was by an intimate partner, with bosses and colleagues in workplaces responsible for 26 per cent, and friends and family for 10 per cent. VAWG was experienced at various times over women's life course. For example, forty-year-old Sofia had experienced the following in London and Brazil: she had been locked up, had her hair pulled, and been beaten, kicked, raped, insulted, harassed, controlled and financially abused by her husband; outside the home, she had been sexually abused by a fellow churchgoer in London.

In Rio, where awareness was more limited, incidence levels were lower. Although the vast majority of those surveyed (76 per cent) stated that VAWG occurs in Maré, only 28 per cent openly stated that they had suffered it. However, when asked about reporting such violence, 38 per cent stated they had experienced it. In addition, women in the area controlled by militias and with the lowest number of NGOs reported the lowest levels, suggesting that they were potentially afraid to discuss it or were less aware. Those most likely to have experienced GBV were aged between thirty and forty-four, were mixed-race or black, had lived all their lives in Maré, had primary levels of schooling and were single or separated. As for the types of GBV suffered, physical violence emerged as the most important (experienced by 51 per cent of women), followed by psychological/emotional violence (42 per cent) and sexual abuse (7 per cent). Intimate partners committed a third of GBV, and only 15 per cent was perpetrated by strangers; the remainder was committed by work colleagues and bosses and friends and family. As in London, women experienced multiple types of violence over their life course. For example, all the women interviewed had experienced various forms of GBV: fifteen had experienced humiliation and psychological violence, fourteen had suffered physical aggression in the form of punches, kicks and knife attacks, nine had been raped or sexually abused, eight had been mistreated in childhood, eight had been socially ostracised, five had experienced attempted murder, four had been financially abused, and three reported sexism and racism.

The breadth, severity and ubiquity of VAWG among Brazilians in London and in Maré highlights how GBV dominates the lives of women in ways that are often ignored by wider society. In the words of Marcia in London: 'I think it's so rare for women to be listened to. Because what

I'm seeing now is that the blame always falls on us.' This also has important implications for understanding women's equitable participation in the city (Peake, 2017) and beyond at a transnational level (McIlwaine and Evans, 2018; McIlwaine and Evans, and 2020).

Spaces of urban VAWG in London and Rio de Janeiro

Central to understanding the relationships between VAWG and a gender equitable right to the city is how GBV plays out across different scales, domains and territories and how cities in turn are situated within wider global relations of structural violence that also mediate and influence the nature of GBV. This section identifies how VAWG is manifested across these multiple spaces and territories of the city in London and Rio de Janeiro. In London, 30 per cent of all GBV occurred in the domestic domain (22 per cent in the victim's home and 8 per cent in someone else's), mainly in the form of IPV (75 per cent of perpetrators), whereas in Maré, almost half of all GBV was in the private arena (47 per cent), again primarily on the form of IPV. This type of violence was often exceptionally severe, usually taking multiple and overlapping forms. In London, for example, Cristina, aged thirty-seven, from São Paulo, experienced a huge range of violence at the hands of her Brazilian husband Roberto. Among a host of abuses, he continually verbally insulted her, strangled her, hit her with knives and scissors and assaulted her sexually. In addition, he stole money from her and imprisoned her in their house, refusing to let her go to work or to church.

Similar stories emerged in Maré. In one very severe case, Victoria spoke of her husband's abuse:

> He would go there and start hitting me, sometimes lying down, asleep. He was pulling at my hair, picking things up to pinch me. He got to the point of urinating on my legs. He already got to the point of throwing my stuff all down the street, my clothes. He got to the point of locking me in the house, at the carnival, so he could leave.

Domestic violence was also perpetrated in public domains of the city by current and former conjugal partners and other family members. In London, Miriam spoke of how her ex-husband followed her everywhere after they split up, continually harassing her in the street and even throwing a brick through the window of her flat. In Maré, Victoria recalled how her husband chased her into the street and ripped her dress while attacking her. Other family members were often perpetrators of violence both within and beyond the home. In London, Camila spoke about how her brother subjected her to constant physical abuse when she was growing up in Bahia: 'I remember a few episodes of him hitting my head on the wall to make me cry.' Teresa from Maré recalled how her brother assaulted her in the street as part of an argument with their father: 'He took the gun and struck the butt in my head. Then he pointed the rifle at my father and wanted to shoot him.'

In terms of GBV in public spaces more broadly, in London the workplace emerged as a major site of violence where almost a quarter of all violence occurred (23 per cent). Much of this was sexual harassment, as discussed by Isabel, a chambermaid in a hotel, who described how a male colleague had attacked her in an empty room, throwing her on the bed and throttling her while sexually assaulting her, before she managed to escape. Beyond the workplace, other public places where GBV occurred included cafés and bars (16 per cent), public transport (10 per cent) and public areas (10 per cent). In Maré, local public spaces (18 per cent) and the streets of the community (10 per cent) were the most commonly identified places where GBV occurred, with only 5 per cent of instances occurring in the workplace and 1 per cent on public transport. The latter might be explained by high levels of women running their own businesses or working at home, and by low levels of public transport use beyond the favela. Yet, as noted above by Teresa, the GBV experienced in public areas of Maré was extremely severe, especially the sexual violence, and intersected with the high levels of generalised urban violence (see also Wilding, 2010 and 2012). For example, Marcela spoke of her experiences as a girl: 'At twelve, I was raped. I was going to school. Close to home itself. A guy came, took me by the arm and there I was raped.' Another woman, Luana, who had been homeless, spoke of sexual assault:

> I have already undergone rape ... In the old days, it was easy to live on the street. Not today. I'm afraid. In the old days, the cops were bad ... They beat, but they did not kill like today.

This raises the issue of fear, which deeply constrains women's freedom to move around (Whitzman, Andrew and Viswanath, 2014), making it imperative that women create strategies to deal with it, such as changing routes and schedules of movement, and 'judicious' choice of clothing (McIlwaine and Moser, 2007). Such forced immobility and limitations on freedom fundamentally undermine women's right to experience the city on an equal footing with men. Also important here are the experiences of LGBTQ+ people, an issue which is often overlooked in these debates. In Maré, Marisa, a transgender woman, spoke in spatial terms about her violent experiences:

> The relationship I have with this space that for a long time in my life was completely aggressive and violent. I'm a transsexual woman. So I was a boy who walked in this community and suffered physical and verbal aggressions from various spaces, more by men and boys.

Gendered institutional violence also manifests itself in the public domain in insidious ways. In Maré, it was explicitly linked with public insecurity. On one hand, the various armed actors in the community perpetrated VAWG, as noted by Luana with reference to the police. Yet other actors such as gang members and drug dealers also committed violence, sometimes as aggression and a further exercise of their territorial power, and at other times as a form of 'protection' in the absence of state security forces willing to support women (see also Moser and McIlwaine, 2004; Wilding, 2014). For instance, Jennifer spoke of how her husband had come into a bar in the favela and hit her in the face, making her fall over. A group of gang members then confronted her husband and kicked him out. While this was a reactive situation, some women actively seek gang members to assist them in the face of lack of enforcement of legal support by the police. Lina discussed how many women feel compelled to turn to extra-judicial forms of 'parallel power' to deal with VAWG:

> I wanted the law to keep him from me, but then I saw that, unfortunately, because I live in a poor community, they do not do what the law asks ... I've heard their [gangs'] way is to kill or some other threat: 'Man, go away and never come back, because if you come and we see you, we'll kill you.'

While the situation in Maré was of endemic gendered institutional violence, gendered institutional violence also occurred in London, albeit in different forms. It usually entailed abuse of women at the hands of state officials, ranging from the police to border force officials. For example, Camila recollected how she was verbally abused by an immigration officer at a London airport:

> After I'd been interviewed for three hours, I was released to go get my luggage. An immigration officer accompanied me into the lift to take me

to where my luggage was. Inside the lift he said, 'Wow, you've got beautiful breasts. Can I touch them?' Something like that. I looked at him and thought, 'I've just arrived, and the harassment has already started?' I told him no and felt afraid inside the lift.

The final arena of perpetration of urban VAWG is the transnational. Indeed, it emerged that experiences of GBV underpinned women's migration from Brazil (usually from the large cities of São Paulo and Rio de Janeiro) to London, with 77 per cent of those in London stating that they had suffered before they moved. Driven by a general desire to improve their lives, many women discussed how they had fled Brazil to escape violent partners or they had moved with perpetrators in the hope that the violence would diminish. Cristina from São Paulo, for example, moved to London in 2009 with her husband, who had previously been violent towards her, in a bid to save their marriage, yet the violence actually increased. However, Cristina noted that she received support from British social services, which she felt was better than that provided back home (see below). Another dimension of transnational urban VAWG in London was human trafficking and forced labour, with several cases of women who had arrived to work and had passports confiscated and/or ended up living in servitude. One woman, Sabrina, went to London to work for a Brazilian family as a nanny. Although the family organised her visa and travel, on arrival they took her passport and made her look after two children, do all the housework and work for her boss, who was employed as a cleaner and a courier, from early morning to late in the evening. Her boss then began to sexually and physically harass her, prompting her to escape, first through some Brazilian friends and then with the help of a migrant organisation. Indeed, among those who experienced GBV in Brazil, more than half (52 per cent) experienced it again in London, while some others encountering it in London for the first time.

Causes of urban VAWG in London and Rio de Janeiro

The underlying causes of VAWG are patriarchal power relations rooted in sociocultural valorisations of the hegemonic power of men and inferiority of women, undergirded by gender inequalities in material conditions (UN Women, 2015). Although the core gender norms are often resilient to change, gender practices can transform in different places, especially across borders as people migrate (McIlwaine, 2010). Indeed, unequal power relations were identified in Maré and London as causing VAWG, with many women acknowledging that misogyny adapts; one woman in a London focus group noted:

> In Brazil, it is all out in the open. It is common to see men humiliating and swearing at women everywhere. It is a cultural thing, the disrespect for women. It happens here too, of course, but this disrespect is disguised.

Yet Brazilian gendered subjectivities also transform in negative ways in relation to how women are intersectionally stereotyped in the UK through complex racialisation and hyper-sexualisation, with many complaining of being thought of as 'easy', 'sexy' or 'sex workers' by British men in particular (see also Beserra, 2005; Datta and McIlwaine, 2014). This shows how gendered violence interrelates in complex ways with structural and symbolic violence, which ultimately also undermines wider wellbeing and health.

As noted above, there are also other wider forms of insecurity that affect the perpetration of VAWG among Brazilians linked to structural violence from a transnational perspective and are rooted in gendered institutional violence (McIlwaine and Evans, 2018; McIlwaine and Evans, 2020). Some of these are generic while others relate specifically to urban living and working. In relation to migrants in London (where the majority of Brazilian migrants are concentrated), one of the most significant relates to insecure immigration status, which can marginalise women survivors of VAWG whose fear of deportation invariably prevents them from seeking help. Their situation is exacerbated further by lack of English-language proficiency and inability to access state support as part of visa restrictions that limit their access to services such as legal support (the 'No Recourse to Public Funds' stipulation: see below; see also Erez, Adelman and Gregory, 2009). As Valentina explained: 'We are far from our country, don't speak the language, don't have the professions that we would have in our country, we don't belong to society, we're very much on the margins.' Immigration status can also be used as a form of gendered power manipulation (Menjívar and Salcido, 2002) in that reporting to border authorities becomes a tool of abuse; as a service provider stated: 'if the woman is in this country "illegally", and the husband is "legal", he will do whatever he wants with her, because she is at his mercy'. Migrant women can also end up in abusive relationships as a result of marrying for immigration documents. Insecure status also exacerbates public VAWG in that it can lead to migrant women's concentration in low-paid urban work such as cleaning and catering, where they face more exploitative conditions than those with residency rights, as noted by a service provider in London: 'if somebody knows [they are undocumented] they can get away with exploiting ... those women are far more vulnerable to other forms of exploitation, domestic exploitation, sexual slavery'. Negotiating the public spaces of the city can also be dangerous for migrant women. As noted above, harassment in workplaces was commonplace, as was abuse on public transport. Migrant women often end up working in jobs in the city that put them in particular danger. For example, contract cleaning takes places early in the morning or late at night, necessitating travel on night buses, where several women reported abuse (McIlwaine, 2015; see also below).

Therefore, while being a migrant in London produces challenges associated with urban marginality that can precipitate VAWG, in Maré, the main risks factors are associated with the institutional and structural violence associated with residing in a marginalised favela with high levels of urban violence, the proliferation of armed groups, the widespread use of firearms and drugs and the deep neglect of the state (Wilding, 2012). Indeed, the state actively generates violence in Maré through the continual police operations which result in death, injury and closure of schools and health centres and which undermine the rights of women and men to participate in the life of the city (see above), as one woman from Maré noted: 'All this has been taken away from us. We were given the right to come and go. This state, these genocidal, murderous rulers, were taking away all this.' While the exact relationships with VAWG are complex (Wilding, 2010), the fact that so many men are involved in everyday violence as perpetrators and victims can lead to higher levels of GBV as men negotiate hegemonic masculinities in a context where violence is often viewed as the norm (Jewkes, Flood and Land, 2015).

The conditions of living and working as a migrant in London related to exploitative urban employment or negotiating public transport at unsociable hours, for example, or as a favela resident in Rio de Janeiro, where urban violence on the part of the state and armed gangs is endemic, can therefore act as specific 'urban-based triggers' (McIlwaine, 2013) which are themselves forms of structural and symbolic violence. While certain spaces within the city become associated with GBV such as workplaces in London and public spaces in the favela, other shared and more generic risk factors emerged. In relation to intimate partner violence, pregnancy, miscarriage, incestuous sexual abuse in childhood and male substance abuse emerged as precipitating factors (Heise and Kotsadam, 2015). In London, for example, Laura had a Portuguese boyfriend who was addicted to crystal meth and who attacked her when under its influence. In Maré, there was a consensus in the focus group of drug-users that GBV was normal but also that it was especially marked in the 'crack scene'. Sexual abuse in childhood was endemic in Brazil and is known to affect the perpetration and experience of VAWG in later life (Jewkes, Flood and Land, 2015). Among the women in London, many had migrated in order to escape such abuse, while others were continuing to struggle to deal with the consequences. Indeed, eight out of twenty-five reported being subjected to some form of incestuous sexual abuse by fathers, uncles and cousins in Brazil before migration. In Maré, child abuse was ubiquitous. In one severe case, a woman, Maria Elisa, spoke of her sexual abuse by a family member when she was six. This person had even burned her private parts so that she would not tell anyone. A few years later and still traumatised, she fled from a small town near to Recife to Maré with her cousins to escape the abuse.

Urban VAWG and a healthy gendered right to the city in London and Rio de Janeiro

To return to Whitzman, Andrew and Viswanath's (2014: 445) notion of women's right to the city, safety is not just the absence of violence and fear but also involves engendering wellbeing and gender equality through 'a place to live, access to livelihoods and active participation in all aspects of public life, from "loitering" in public space to decision making about public resources'. Yet it is crucial that this is assessed across diverse scales and spaces from the body to the home, community and city and transnationally, and that the causes are acknowledged as being rooted in deep-seated gendered power relations and structural violence. Indeed, a gendered right to the city encompasses the intersections between private and public relationships free from GBV that are sustained through a range of material conditions (Datta, 2016), that stretch across all these spaces in ways which are intricately linked with health and wellbeing. In the London context, health problems caused by

VAWG were identified by all of the service providers as a major issue. One organisation working specifically with Latin American women noted that among 133 Brazilian users between 2013 and 2017, physical and mental health problems accounted for 25 per cent of their consultations, much of which were linked with violence, with another 20 per cent seeking support in relation to sex work where, again, health problems were prominent (Evans and McIlwaine, 2017). Demand for counselling and psychotherapy was extremely high within this organisation, which reported long waiting lists. Indeed, mental health problems appeared to be endemic among migrant women. Cristina spoke of the damage to her mental health and its consequences:

> Everything leaves a scar. I get terrible migraines every time I speak about this, either before or after. I start throwing up and I spend four days bedridden, in the dark, wearing earplugs and an eye mask because I can't hear any noise. This causes me problems at work, my boss has pulled me up on it, complaining that I only work eighteen hours per week and that I need to try harder.

A representative from another organisation working specifically on providing health services for sex workers, including Brazilian women, reported how this was invariably related with gendered violence:

> So very often people come here [for] sexual reproductive health, and [then] we find that other things are going on, such as sexual assault, rape, DV (domestic violence) … The commonest violence that we see here in the clinic is women who've experienced violence in their work setting, and that can be sexual violence, or non-sexual, so it can be that people are actually robbing them of money or goods, and/or sexual violence. They are either people who have been raped or sexually assaulted. And also … customers come to see them and after one service, try something else, which often is rape or sexual assault.

In Maré, as discussed above, the effects of everyday violence and its intersection with GBV fundamentally affected women's ability to walk freely in the streets of the community and the wider city of Rio. Fear was insidious, limiting mobility and creating silences, as noted by Mariah:

> I watched a lot. I close my eyes, like this … I've seen many things happen and I could not speak because you cannot speak … What can you talk about? We cannot. There's a man beating a woman. Even if I say so, that woman does not react, or if she reacts, she will be against me.

Yet there are also feminised paradoxes of city life for women in relation to VAWG that provide at least some potential for more gender equity, however limited (Chant and McIlwaine, 2016). To return to the notion of the city as an arena where patriarchal strictures are less marked than in rural areas, similar flexibilities in gender identities pertain when migrants move internationally to cities of the global north (McIlwaine and Carlisle, 2011). While they are certainly not clear-cut in either instance (McIlwaine, 2013), and despite alarming levels of gendered violence in London and Maré, some women in both places spoke of reduced tolerance of such violence. Just as Maria Elisa had fled a small town near Recife and moved to Maré because of incestuous sexual abuse, some women in London spoke of fleeing Brazil because of VAWG and of finding the UK more supportive of women who experienced GBV. Indeed, when women in London were asked to compare the incidence of VAWG across the two contexts, some thought that it was the same or worse (44 per cent), while 43 per cent felt that it was less frequent. When reflecting on the differences, Sofia stated:

> I feel that in Brazil violence against women is more common, people think it's not such a bad thing. Here I have the feeling it's seen as a serious crime. I can see this difference very clearly. However, when you are foreigner here, things are more difficult.

Indeed, despite many instances of neglect in London, many women spoke of support from the police and organisations that was absent in Brazil. Carolina, who spoke of her experience of reporting IPV, stated: 'Here, if you call the police, they take action immediately. I have a gadget with me, it's like a little mobile phone. When I reported him for the first time, they gave me this.'

These differences are reflected in levels of reporting and disclosure of GBV in both contexts, in that 56 per cent of women never reported it in London (to either friends, family or formal channels) in comparison to 65 per cent in Maré. The main reason for this in London was that they thought that nothing would be done about it, together with a lack of information, and in Maré, that they did not think the violence was serious. It appears that while GBV is certainly widespread everywhere, with higher levels of tolerance in Maré than in London, women perceive variations in tolerance and support, especially if they are migrants. Urban living does not therefore uniformly put women at risk of experiencing VAWG. While there are urban-specific causes underpinning

VAWG, there is also less tolerance of it and more support for those who have suffered in London.

Conclusions

This chapter has explored the role of VAWG in the configuration of healthy feminised urban futures from the perspective of Brazilians living in London and those residing in a marginalised favela community in Rio de Janeiro. It reinforces calls for a healthy gendered right to the city to be acknowledged much more explicitly in academic and policy debates (Peake, 2017). In turn, it argues for the importance of explicitly taking VAWG into account in such debates, especially in relation to its role in undermining gender equity and wellbeing in the city. The empirical findings from London and Rio de Janeiro show that the endemic and extensive nature of VAWG has a host of deleterious outcomes for women's health, productivity and wellbeing, which make these calls ever more urgent. In both places, multidimensional forms of VAWG occurred across private and public domains of the city, with the workplace being especially important in London and the street and public space being especially significant in Rio de Janeiro, and various types emerging at the transnational scale associated with the migration process between Brazil and the UK. While the causes of VAWG were rooted in insidious unequal gendered power relations which were resilient across borders, these intersected with urban-specific forms of structural violence that undermined people's wellbeing and health (DeVerteuil, 2015). In London, these revolved around specific types of urban employment in cleaning and sex work that are highly exploitative, especially when women have insecure immigration status and low levels of language competency. In Rio, everyday violence associated with state security forces and armed gangs could exacerbate VAWG in the favelas. Yet, while levels of gendered violence are often higher in cities (McIlwaine 2013), the paradox of residing in certain urban areas can mean that women may be more aware of what GBV entails and more able to secure support, especially when dealing with the health consequences. Yet this should not distract from the importance of addressing VAWG as a major threat to gender-equitable and healthy feminised urban futures and especially the underlying gendered and structural power relations that undergird it in context-specific ways.

Acknowledgements

We would like to thank the British Economic and Social Research Council (ESRC) and Newton Fund, which funded the research on which this chapter is based (grant ES/N013247/1), as well as our partners in the research, the People's Palace Projects, the Latin American Women's Rights Service in London and Redes da Maré in Rio de Janeiro. In addition, we are grateful to those involved at various stages of the project including Paul Heritage, Rosana Morgado, Joana Garcia, Gisele Martins and Isabela Souza, Aline Littlejohn, Renata Peppl, Raquel Roldanus-Dias, Rosie Hunter and Thiago Jesus. We are also grateful to Michael Keith and Andreza A. De Souza Santos for their helpful comments on an earlier draft.

References

Bapat, M., and Agarwal, I. (2003). Our needs, our priorities: Women and men from the slums of Mumbai and Pune talk about their need for water and sanitation. *Environment and Urbanization*, 15(2): 71–86.

Beserra, B. (2005). From Brazilians to Latinos? Racialization and Latinidad in the making of Brazilian carnival in Los Angeles. *Latino Studies*, 3: 53–75.

Bondi, L., and Christie, H. (2003). Working out the urban: Gender relations and the city. In G. Bridge and S. Watson (eds), *A companion to the city*, 293–305. Oxford: Blackwell.

Bradshaw, S. (2013). Women's decision-making in rural and urban households in Nicaragua. *Environment and Urbanization*, 25: 81–94.

Chant, S. (2013). Cities through a 'gender lens': A golden 'urban age' for women in the global south? *Environment and Urbanization*, 25: 9–29.

Chant, S., and McIlwaine, C. (2016). *Cities, slums and gender in the global south: Towards a feminised urban future*. London: Routledge.

Datta, A. (2016). The intimate city: Violence, gender and ordinary life in Delhi slums. *Urban Geography*, 37: 323–42.

Datta, K., and McIlwaine, C. (2014). Negotiating masculinised migrant rights and everyday citizenship in a global city: Brazilian men in London. In A. Gorman-Murray and P. Hopkins (eds), *Masculinities and place*, 93–108. Aldershot: Ashgate.

DeVerteuil, G. (2015). Conceptualizing violence for health and medical geography. *Social Science and Medicine*, 133: 216–22.

Dominguez, S., and Menjívar, C. (2014). Beyond individual and visible acts of violence: A framework to examine the lives of women in low-income neighborhoods. *Women's Studies International Forum*, 44: 184–95.

Erez, E., Adelman, M., and Gregory, C. (2009). Intersections of immigration and domestic violence: Voices of battered immigrant women. *Feminist Criminology*, 4: 32–56.

Esser, D. (2014). Security scales: Spectacular and endemic violence in post-invasion Kabul, Afghanistan. *Environment and Urbanization*, 26: 373–88.

Evans, Y., Dias, G., Martins, A. Jr, Souza, A., and Tonhati, T. (2015). *Diversidade de oportunidades: Brasileiros em Londres*. London: Grupo de Estudos Sobre Brasileiros no Reino Unido.

Evans, Y., and McIlwaine, C. (2017). Supporting Brazilian women in London: Service provision for survivors of violence against women and girls (VAWG). London: Queen Mary University of London.

Evans, Y., Tonhati, T., Dias, G., Brightwell, G., Sheringham, O., and Souza, A. (2011). Brazilians in London: A report. *Canadian Journal of Latin American and Caribbean Studies*, 36: 235–48.

Fenster, T. (2005). The right to the gendered city: Different formations of belonging in everyday life. *Journal of Gender Studies*,14: 217–31.

Guimarães, M.C., and Pedroza, R.L.S. (2015). Violência contra a mulher: Problematizando definições teóricas, filosóficas e jurídicas. *Psicologia e Sociedade*, 27: 256–66.

Heise, L. (1998). Violence against women: An integrated, ecological framework. *Violence against Women*, 4(3): 262–90.

Heise, L., Ellsberg, M., and Gottmoeller, M. (2002). A global overview of gender-based violence. *International Journal of Gynaecology and Obstetrics*, 78: S5–S14.

Heise, L., and Kotsadam, A. (2015). Cross-national and multilevel correlates of partner violence. *Lancet Global*, 3: 332–40.

Hindin, M.J., and Adair, L.S. (2002). Who's at risk? Factors associated with intimate partner violence in the Philippines. *Social Science and Medicine*, 55: 1385–99.

Jewkes, R., Flood, M., and Land, J. (2015). From work with men and boys to changes of social norms and reduction of inequalities in gender relations. *Lancet*, 385(9977): 1580–9.

Kiss, L., Schraiber, L.B., Heise, L., Zimmerman, C., Gouveia, N., and Watts, C. (2012). Gender-based violence and socioeconomic inequalities: Does living in more deprived neighbourhoods increase women's risk of intimate partner violence? *Social Science and Medicine*, 74: 1172–9.

Krenzinger, M., Sousa Silva, E., McIlwaine, C., and Heritage, P. (eds) (2018). *Dores que liberam*. Rio de Janeiro: Attis.

McIlwaine, C. (2010). Migrant machismos: Exploring gender ideologies and practices among Latin American migrants in London from a multi-scalar perspective. *Gender, Place and Culture*, 17: 281–300.

McIlwaine, C. (2013). Urbanisation and gender-based violence: Exploring the paradoxes in the global south. *Environment and Urbanization*, 25: 65–79.

McIlwaine, C. (2015). Legal Latins: Creating webs and practices of immigration status among Latin American migrants in London. *Journal of Ethnic and Migration Studies*, 41(3): 493–511.

McIlwaine, C. (2016). Gender-based violence and assets in just cities: Triggers and transformation. In C. Moser (ed.), *Gender, asset accumulation and just cities*, 150–63. London: Routledge.

McIlwaine, C., and Bunge, D. (2016). *Towards visibility: The Latin American community in London*. London: Trust for London.

McIlwaine, C., and Carlisle, F. (2011). Gender transformations and gender-based violence among Latin American migrants in London. In C. McIlwaine (ed.), *Cross-border migration among Latin Americans*, 157–74. New York: Palgrave Macmillan.

McIlwaine, C., and Evans, Y. (2018). *We can't fight in the dark: Violence against women and girls (VAWG) among Brazilians in London*. London: King's College London.

McIlwaine, C., and Evans, Y. (2020). Urban violence against women and girls (VAWG) in transnational perspective: Reflections from Brazilian women in London. *International Development Planning Review*, 42(1): 93–112.

McIlwaine, C., and Moser, C. (2007). Living in fear: How the urban poor perceive violence, fear and insecurity. In K. Koonings and D. Kruijt (eds), *Fractured cities: Social exclusion, urban violence and contested spaces in Latin America*, 117–37. London: Zed.

Menjívar, C., and Salcido, O. (2002). Immigrant women and domestic violence: Common experiences in different countries. *Gender and Society*, 16: 898–920.

Michau, L., Horn, J., Bank, A., Dutt, M., and Zimmerman, C. (2015). Prevention of violence against women and girls: Lessons from practice. *Lancet*, 385: 1672–84.

Moser, C. (ed.) (2016). *Gender, asset accumulation and just cities*. London: Routledge.

Moser, C. (2017). Gender transformation in a new global urban agenda: Challenges for Habitat III and beyond. *Environment and Urbanization*, 29: 221–36.

Moser, C., and McIlwaine, C. (2004). *Encounters with violence in Latin America*. London: Routledge.

Moser, C., and McIlwaine, C. (2014). New frontiers in twenty-first century urban conflict and violence. *Environment and Urbanization*, 26: 331–44.

Pain, R. (2014). Everyday terrorism: Connecting domestic violence global terrorism. *Progress in Human Geography*, 38: 531–50.

Peake, L. (2016). The twenty-first century quest for feminism and the global urban. *International Journal of Urban and Regional Research*, 40: 219–27.

Peake, L. (2017). Feminism and the urban. In J.R. Short (ed.), *A Research Agenda for Cities*, 82–97. Cheltenham: Edward Elgar.

Peake, L., and Rieker, M. (2013). Rethinking feminist interventions into the urban. In L. Peake and M. Rieker, *Rethinking feminist interventions into the urban*, 1–22. London: Routledge.

Philo, C. (2017). Less-than-human geographies. *Political Geography*, 60: 256–58.

Rights of Women (2013). *Evidencing domestic violence: A barrier to family law legal aid*. Rights of Women, London, https://rightsofwomen.org.uk/wp-content/uploads/2014/10/Evidencing-DV-a-barrier-2013.pdf (last accessed 20 February 2020).

Sousa Silva, E. (2017). *The Brazilian army's occupation of Maré*. Rio de Janeiro: Redes da Maré.

Tankel, Y. (2011). Reframing 'safe cities for women': Feminist articulations in Recife. *Development*, 54(3): 352–57.

UN-Habitat (2006). *The State of the World's Cities 2006/2007*. London: Earthscan.

UN Women (2015). *A framework to underpin action to prevent violence against women*. New York: UN Women.

Vacchelli, E., Kathrecha, P., and Gyte, N. (2015). Is it really just the cuts? *Feminist Review*, 109: 180–9.

Vacchelli, E., and Kofman, E. (2018). Towards an inclusive and gendered right to the city. *Cities*, 26: 1–3.

Watts, C., and Zimmerman, C. (2002). Violence against women: Global scope and magnitude. *Lancet*, 359(9313): 1232–7.

Whitzman, C., Andrew, C., and Viswanath, K. (2014). Partnerships for women's safety in the city: 'Four legs for a good table'. *Environment and Urbanization*, 26: 443–56.

WHO (2002). *World report on violence and health*. Geneva: WHO.

WHO (2013). *Global and regional estimates of violence against women: prevalence and health effects of intimate partner violence and non-partner sexual violence*. Geneva: WHO.

Wilding, P. (2010). New violence: Silencing women's experiences in the favelas of Brazil. *Journal of Latin American Studies*, 42: 719–47.

Wilding, P. (2012). *Negotiating boundaries: Gender, violence and transformation in Brazil*. Basingstoke: Palgrave.

Wilding, P. (2014). Gendered meanings and everyday experiences of violence in urban Brazil. *Gender, Place and Culture*, 21(2): 228–43.

4

Understanding the relationships between wellbeing and mobility in the unequal city: the case of community initiatives promoting cycling and walking in São Paulo and London

Tim Schwanen and Denver V. Nixon

Whether city living contributes to people's wellbeing is a question that both is topical and, in the Western tradition, goes back to at least Ancient Greece. It is topical because of the broader happiness turn (Ahmed, 2010) and the steady increases in urbanisation on the planetary scale (Satterthwaite, 2007). The question can be answered in many different ways, although quantitative analysis regressing one or more indicators of subjectively experienced wellbeing onto a host of measures of opulence, social networks, the built environment, population composition and so on tends to prevail in the recent academic literature (Ballas, 2013; Okuliz-Kozaryn, 2015; Winters and Li, 2017). Other research has considered how everyday time use in the city, including transport, shapes wellbeing (De Vos et al., 2013; Schwanen and Wang, 2014; Birenboim, 2018). Work along these lines typically understands wellbeing as a subjective state that inheres in individuals and can be measured quantitatively (Atkinson, 2013).

This mode of analysis is in keeping with the neoliberal governmental regimes under which wellbeing has become a major object of intervention (Binkley, 2014). Questions can nevertheless be raised about its usefulness in situations of extreme inequality between people in terms of wealth, health, resources and entitlements as they exist – and, if anything, seem to be increasing – in many cities across the world. This is not least because adaptive preferences may make poor and other disadvantaged people inclined to accept situations and inequalities that can be argued to be objectively unjust or oppressive (Sen, 2008). It is also not clear whether prevailing modes of quantitative analysis of subjectively experienced wellbeing can offer adequate insight into the collective dimensions of wellbeing in the city, and into the ways in which differences in wellbeing between people in a city or between different moments in a given person's life emerge and unfold.

In this chapter, we therefore engage with different traditions of conceptualising and examining wellbeing to understand some of the relationships between everyday mobility and wellbeing in deeply unequal cities with a specific focus on disadvantaged social groups. A version of the Capabilities Approaches (CAs) originally developed by Amartya Sen and colleagues (Sen, 1999; Robeyns, 2017) plays a prominent role in our analysis. That version is, however, extended and amalgamated with insights from relational, process-based perspectives on wellbeing from Human Geography (Smith and Reid, 2018) according to which wellbeing can be understood as emerging from practices and relations in particular time-spaces and referring to closely interrelated, individualised experiences and capabilities to be and become otherwise. Since forms of mobility often play a central part in those experiences and capabilities, sociological thinking on motility – potential mobility (Kaufmann, 2002; see below) – is also used. We thus begin to elaborate a revised approach to capabilities in an attempt to shed light on how wellbeing is generated in time-spaces that are always differentiated and differentiating.

In empirical terms, our discussion draws on research conducted in the deeply unequal cities of São Paulo and London and concentrating on the role of citizen-led initiatives to support cycling and walking among people in poor or otherwise deprived neighbourhoods of both cities. This focus may seem unduly narrow, but we argue that the initiatives' practices have an infrastructural relationship to wellbeing as relationally generated experience and capabilities. This is because, in all their heterogeneity, the initiatives seek to actively overcome transport disadvantage – lack of access, knowledge, skills, aspiration, autonomy and/or influence over institutionalised policy and governance with regard to transport and everyday mobility – of specific social groups and broader socio-spatial inequalities in the neoliberalised city, often through prefigurative politics (Yates, 2015). Moreover, walking and cycling are, on balance, the most just forms of everyday urban mobility.

Even if both are increasingly co-opted by entrepreneurial and speculative urban regeneration efforts, restrictions on access to them and their imprints on cities (air pollution, greenhouse gases, noise, congestion, differentiation between haves and have-nots, evictions and displacement) tend to be considerably lower for them than for public transport and private automobiles.

The remainder of this chapter is in four parts. We begin with a brief discussion of wellbeing and mobility as concepts before summarising our understanding of their interrelationships. This is followed by a summary description of the empirical research, after which we critically explore how citizen-led initiatives to promote cycling and walking contribute to wellbeing in deprived urban communities. The chapter ends with some propositions.

Core concepts and analytical framework

Wellbeing

The term 'wellbeing' is easily used but often poorly defined, and conceptualisations abound in both popular discourse and the academic literature. There is evidence to suggest that, at least in the Western world, understandings of wellbeing have become increasingly centred on the individual under the influence of neoliberalism and the rise of the 'psy-sciences' (Ahmed, 2010; Binkley, 2014). Much contemporary research and policy discourse therefore understands wellbeing as a subjective and hedonic state that inheres in individuals (Atkinson, 2013). On this account, wellbeing is about what individuals feel: how satisfied, happy, free from pain and so forth they are in general or at a specific point in time. This is the kind of wellbeing that is imagined, measured and analysed by the 'science' of wellbeing (Diener, 2000) and increasingly dominant in transport and urban studies research.

The science of wellbeing is, however, not restricted to hedonic understandings of wellbeing as eudaimonic conceptions have steadily gained ground over the past decades. Drawing on Aristotle's writings, psychologists have argued that wellbeing is not about the maximisation of pleasure but about flourishing – the realisation of one's *daimon* or true potential, as well as fulfilment and meaning in life. Wellbeing, in this imagination, still inheres in individuals as a state (Ryan and Deci, 2001; Ryff and Singer, 2008). The most widely considered states in this context relate to personal growth, autonomy, social relationships and relatedness, competence, environmental mastery and self-acceptance. While offering a more textured and complex understanding of wellbeing than most hedonic approaches, the thinking by eudaimonic psychologists has been criticised for its paternalism, ethnocentric universalisation of Euro-American conceptions of human subjectivity and experience, and reduction of wellbeing to quantifiable and discrete components (Atkinson, 2013; Smith and Reid, 2018).

Many other conceptualisations of wellbeing exist, and a full overview is beyond this chapter. Two, however, deserve special mention. Linked to the above eudaimonic perspective are the CAs that have emerged in the wake of Amartya Sen's work on development and freedom (Sen, 1999; Robeyns, 2017). Different CAs come with markedly different ontological assumptions, for instance in terms of commitment to individualism and universalism, and ethical implications (Robeyns, 2017). Sen's own version is adamant in its rejection of conceptualising wellbeing in terms of resources (including wealth) and happiness or other subjective experiences. Wellbeing is rather about the capabilities available to individuals: the positive freedom to achieve certain activities and states of being. He distinguishes between functionings – actually achieved activities and states of being – and capabilities, which represent real opportunities or potentials. When discussing wellbeing, Sen tends to privilege capabilities over functionings, stressing that the conversion of capabilities into actual functionings is mediated by all kinds of personal and social factors, from previous functionings such as acquired skills and remembered experiences to policy outcomes, economic structures and discourses (Sen, 1999; Clark, 2005; Robeyns, 2017). Thus having a bicycle available (resource) is not enough to contribute to an individual's wellbeing and freedom to engage in functionings elsewhere in physical space if they have not learnt how to cycle (skill) or are discouraged by first-hand experience of traffic accidents (functioning), by road designs privileging motorised vehicles, or discourses equating cycling with backwardness (social factors).

While Sen's CA is, for some, 'broad enough to capture all aspects of human wellbeing' (Clark, 2005: 1340), questions can be raised over its marginalisation of experience, its account of how capabilities come into existence and its individualism. For Clark (2005), hedonic and eudaimonic experiences should be given more credit as valuable functionings than Sen tends to grant them. This is because such experiences are not only a means to an end, facilitating the achievement of other functionings – as Sen has recognised – but also intrinsically valuable constituents of a good life and thus ends in themselves. The argument implies that capabilities, practices and experiences are closely interrelated and need to be understood as co-constitutive of wellbeing.

Sen's texts can induce rather mechanistic accounts of how capabilities come into existence and differ across populations, using econometrics to correlate static indicators of resources, personal and social factors, and capabilities. However, more relational accounts avoiding the specification of *a priori* factors or processes that generate capabilities and their conversion into functionings are also possible. The latter insist on the need to engage with and explore specific situations in particular times and places (Smith and Reid, 2018; White, 2017).

Such accounts can also throw into question the idea that capabilities are ultimately situated at the level of the individual, even if 'their realisation [requires] action by a group or a collectivity' (Robeyns, 2017: 117). This is because relational accounts recognise that capabilities and functionings may be individually experienced but produced by, and emerging from, assemblages of practices, technological artefacts, materiality, discourse and atmospheres (see also Smith and Reid, 2018; White, 2017). Those accounts can foreground that wellbeing, and thus capabilities, happen as events produced and experienced as part of specific times and spaces – time-spaces.

The final conceptualisation of wellbeing discussed in this chapter, then, gathers together a range of process-based, relational accounts of wellbeing as the emergent, space- and time-specific outcome of relations between not only people but also objects, material landscapes, values, discourses and atmospheres as active agents (Smith and Reid, 2018). One of the most helpful outcomes of this style of thinking about wellbeing and its generation is a heuristic classification of how spatial, or rather tempo-spatial, and dynamic constellations of heterogeneous elements – assemblages (Deleuze and Guattari, 1987) – in cities and beyond can enhance wellbeing (Fleuret and Atkinson, 2007):

1. *Time-spaces of capability* that cultivate the capabilities of interest to Sen, particularly for those who suffer comparative disadvantages, such as the stigmatised or disabled;
2. *Time-spaces of social integration* that harness opportunities for people to form networks and relationships with human and non-human others;

3. *Time-spaces of security* that reduce all kinds of risk relating to, for example, traffic injury, violence and other forms of oppression; and
4. *Therapeutic time-spaces* that promote healing, restoration and recuperation, for instance from stress, air pollution and obesogenic and car-dominated environments.

Mobility

As a concept, mobility is as polysemous as wellbeing is (Kaufmann, Bergman and Joye, 2004; Urry, 2007). Most definitions refer to realised or actual movement in social or physical space, such as upward social mobility, migration, residential relocation, tourism and daily commuting or trips for shopping, care or leisure. Yet for authors like Hägerstrand (1970) and Kaufmann (2002), a focus on actual movement is inadequate for an understanding of either how the urban fabric and societal processes enable and constrain mobility, or what the wider consequences of mobility are. Kaufmann and colleagues instead advocate an orientation towards motility: 'the capacity of entities (e.g. goods, information or persons) to be mobile in social and geographic space, or as the way in which entities access and appropriate the capacity for socio-spatial mobility according to their circumstances' (Kaufmann, Bergman and Joye, 2004: 750).

There are parallels here with the concept of accessibility, which is widely used in geography, transport and urban planning literatures to denote 'the potential of opportunities for interaction' (Hansen, 1959: 73) or the 'ease of reaching goods, services, activities and destinations' (Litman, 2017: 6). Nevertheless, for Flamm and Kaufmann (2006), the relationship between individuals or social groups and space is different in both concepts: in accessibility the emphasis is on the opportunities a given spatial configuration offers to individuals, whereas in motility the relation is more two-sided, and individuals or social groups are more active agents.

For Kaufman and colleagues, motility has three interdependent constituents (Kaufmann, Bergman and Joye, 2004):

1. *Access* – the portfolio of mobilities rendered possible by place-specific and time-varying conditions created by transport and communication networks and services, the built environment and urban planning, socio-economic processes, discourses and cultural values, and so on;

2. *Competencies* – the embodied operational (i.e. how things work), navigational (i.e. where things are), temporal (i.e. scheduling) and kinaesthetic (i.e. motor skills) abilities that make particular mobilities using specific technologies and infrastructures possible; and
3. *Cognitive appropriation* – how individuals or social groups consider, deem appropriate and select certain possibilities on the basis of needs, aspirations, motives, values, understandings and habits. The term refers to how individuals and groups act upon access and competencies.

Kaufmann and colleagues use the adjective 'cognitive' consistently in relation to appropriation but this seems unnecessarily restrictive, especially when insights from scholarship on affect are considered according to which non-conscious sensation and embodied perception are much faster and condition conscious thought and experience (Thrift, 2008). Since cognitive appropriation is only one type of appropriation by individuals, we prefer to refer to appropriation in the remainder of this chapter.

The wellbeing-mobility nexus

Relational, process-based perspectives on wellbeing extend and refract Sen's version of the CA. Not only can they foreground the entwined, rather than separated, nature of capabilities and experiences; they can also understand wellbeing 'as *happening*, as always *becoming*, and so always incomplete' (White, 2017: 124; emphasis in original). Hedonic and eudaimonic experiences and capabilities may be individualised into a specific human body and mind, but they are collectively and continuously generated in wider assemblages, from which individuals cannot easily be abstracted in thought and research practices, if dynamics and changes in wellbeing are to be understood. Experiences and capabilities emerge from practices involving interactions with heterogeneous elements – human and non-human – in particular time-spaces. Those time-spaces stand in an infrastructural relationship to experiences and capabilities: they harness and cultivate certain experiences, practices and capabilities, while at the same time making others less likely, sometimes excluding those others altogether and thus producing ambiguous outcomes (as illustrated below).

Mobility is often key to the experiences and capabilities cultivated in time-spaces of wellbeing, particularly in cities where everyday practices are spatially and temporally sorted and inequalities in resources, functionings and capabilities are often rampant. As discussed above, mobility as actual movement is a functioning and a capability that opens up and facilitates the achievement of other functionings. Yet exactly how mobility operates as both functioning and capability remains opaque in CAs, even when amplified by relational and process-based perspectives on wellbeing as an entwined becoming of experience and capability. This is where the thinking on motility is useful. It can highlight how access, competencies and appropriation – themselves continuously and relationally generated in and through interactions and relations within assemblages – are important to the formation of capabilities and their conversion into actual acts and experiences of movement and thus particular functionings and further capabilities. Exactly how access, competences and appropriation emerge, interact and open up functionings and capabilities is an empirical question to which we turn now.

Research in São Paulo and London

The empirical research used for this chapter seeks to address questions about the extent to which citizen-led (rather than state-led) initiatives to promote cycling and walking can accelerate a transition towards more sustainable and just urban mobility systems in unequal cities in the Majority and Minority Worlds. São Paulo and London are the respective cases. Both cities are fast growing in terms of population and dominant in their national economies yet characterised by deep inequalities. São Paulo is the world's ninth most unequal city when the Palma Ratio, the richest 10 per cent's share of income divided by the share of the poorest 40 per cent, is considered (Razvadauskas, 2017). With 1.7 in London (Tinson et al., 2017) that ratio is much lower than São Paulo's 4.8 but still large, particularly for a Minority World context. For some time now, both cities have also been national and continental leaders in pro-cycling policies (segregated bicycle infrastructure, bicycle-sharing schemes and promotional campaigns) advocated by mayoral governments. However, whereas car ownership and use has peaked in London (Metz, 2015), it continues to grow in São Paulo (SINDIPEÇAS and ABIPEÇAS, 2017). It also seems that government policies to encourage cycling and walking are not effectively reaching out to all social groups in both cities. Patterns of social and spatial differentiation in this regard differ between the cities because of their respective historical evolution, physical layout and distribution of social privilege.

Initiatives promoting cycling and walking and specifically targeting disadvantaged individuals and social groups were identified differently in São Paulo and London because of differences in data availability. For London, we used government data on walking and cycling levels and on multiple deprivation to select specific deprived wards (the primary electoral divisions in England) with extensive cycling and/or walking across Greater London. The selected wards lie in four different boroughs (local authority districts), two in Inner London and two in Outer London. Citizen-led initiatives in the identified wards were enumerated through internet searches, local key informants and multiple site visits. Twenty-six initiative leaders and staff willing to participate in the study were interviewed, alongside thirteen beneficiaries. Using snowballing techniques we recruited a further five interviewees involved in, or with knowledge of, similar initiatives across other parts of London.

Since similarly detailed, current and robust geo-spatial data on cycling and walking were unavailable for São Paulo, a list of citizen-led walking and cycling initiatives across the city was compiled using internet searches, local key informants and Como Anda's (2017) national survey. Invited to participate in the study were organisations on this list that run initiatives focused either on deprived neighbourhoods, which were identified using local government data, or on specific disadvantaged groups, such as people with physical disabilities. Twenty-five leaders and staff, plus eight beneficiaries, of citizen-led initiatives were interviewed, as were five intermediaries and government staff members. All interviews in both cities were semi-structured in nature; most were audio-recorded and transcribed, and notes were taken in instances where recording was refused. Just over half of the interviews were conducted in Portuguese; English was used in the remainder when the participants felt comfortable communicating in that language. Resulting texts have been read repeatedly and coded thematically.

Initiatives included walking and cycling groups; bicycle repair training; bicycle riding instruction; the provision of street furniture; the provision of navigational aids; temporary street closures; and pathway, staircase and bicycle-path improvements. The initiatives tended to cater to members of specific disadvantaged social groups, such as those with disabilities, members of cultural and religious minorities, refugees and asylum seekers, women and gender-variant people, low-income residents of deprived neighbourhoods, children and older people. Despite minimal financial and human resources, most originators, leaders and staff sought to run their initiatives on the basis of visions of a more socially just and environmentally responsible society. They attempted to enact these visions, and create new collective norms, through prefiguratively 'leading by example' and experimental interventions in existing transport regimes and political frames (Yates, 2015). Several differences existed between initiatives in São Paulo and London, including a greater focus on walking and following of political tides (campaigning during administrations that promote cycling and walking, and a stronger do-it-yourself or do-it-together orientation at times of conflict and disagreement with local government) in the former city.

Cultivating the potential to walk or cycle

Wellbeing, mobility and space interconnected

Before considering how access, competencies and appropriation interact in the case of the citizen-led initiatives to promote cycling and walking, we begin with a more general discussion of how wellbeing as a combination of capabilities, practices and experiences is closely interconnected with mobility and space. Study participants in both São Paulo and London spoke about their interconnection in various ways and from different perspectives. For some, like Antonio below, overcoming automobility – the landscapes, materialities, practices and institutions centred on the private car – is key to the creation of a more equal and humane city, enabling greater capability sets for everybody instead of only the richer social groups. He articulates a well-rehearsed argument from mobilities scholarship across the social sciences that fast and mechanised forms of mobility, including automobility, are relational in the sense that the mobility of some is achieved through the immobilisation of others (Urry, 2007). The character that the urban fabric – the constellation of the built environment plus social relations, institutions and practices – acquires under automobility plays a key mediating role in that process of socially selective immobilisation and de-capacitation. Cycling, he argues, is more democratic as it opens up not only the capability, even the right, to move but also particular livelihoods to a wider range of people:

So, if people don't have opportunities to access schools, health, activities, the streets, and leisure, this country, this city is not well developed. So, we try to use the bicycle as a tool to enlarge the opportunities and the freedom so people get this kind of thing, but indirectly. The first one is the right to go and come.[1] The second is to learn a profession as a mechanic, a bicycle mechanic, or to work as a bike messenger or a cycle tourist guide, different kinds of professions to which the bicycle is related. We also hope to promote a more humane city with public space shared in a more democratic way. When the streets are made for cars, this is not democratic because they are only for people who have money to buy and use the car, and there is no space for everybody. (Antonio, initiator of a cycling promotion organisation, São Paulo)

Cycling's indirect eudaimonic benefit of opening up particular livelihoods aligns with other research in cities across the Majority World demonstrating how transport is an important source of employment, particularly for young adult men with few educational qualifications (Schwanen, 2018).

The notion that the character of urban space is a barrier to experiences of flourishing and happiness and capability formation was a recurrent theme across interviews. Consider Phoebe and Madalena, whose experiences and positionalities are significantly different. The former comments on the privatisation and commodification of spaces in London where children can enjoy themselves, nurture relationships and learn, whereas the latter reflects on how the capability to walk is empowering and helps to mitigate the unfamiliarity and social atomisation induced by automobility and fear of crime in the north-east of São Paulo:

[The initiative provides] a common, public space. It's really crucial. And I think there's an understanding with all these walking projects and cycling projects and all of the wellbeing, all of the things that come under wellbeing, public space is a really big part of that. This is a public space, it's a drop in. Do you know how many times when we first opened children would come in – and it makes me cry even thinking about it – and asking how much it was? How much to come in and play? What? Yeah. The fact that the expectation is already that they're going to have to pay to go somewhere nice, and that's … And free space, it's amazing, children will go and hang out anywhere that's free. (Phoebe, co-leader of an organisation providing youth cycling training and maintenance as well as a children's playground, London)

> [Walking] means the freedom to do my daily tasks with ease … [The initiative] is a creative, accessible, and enjoyable movement in which to participate. It showed me how important is to think about our wellbeing, and that we can overcome our difficulties … our neighbourhood, and surrounding neighbourhoods, have many stories to tell and places to explore … The friends we make on each walk, the community benefits from these connections. (Madalena, participant in an organised group walk initiative, São Paulo)

Indeed, our analysis reinforces the idea that actual and potential cycling and walking can increase wellbeing for disadvantaged individuals in highly unequal cities owing to the resulting immediate experiences and the capabilities and functionings – activities and contacts at destinations, livelihoods, and so forth – that are opened up. Also important are the indirect, higher-order and longer-term benefits: the cycling and walking by some and the urban fabrics conducive to cycling and walking multiply and extend to others opportunities to flourish and feel well. Currently highly unequal cities may through this become more liveable, equitable and enjoyable.

Access

The quotations from Antonio, Phoebe and Madalena all point out the significance of access, mobilities on foot and by bicycle made possible for specific groups of somehow disadvantaged individuals. They refer to, respectively, inhabitants of São Paulo unable to afford or use a car, children across London and people living in a north-eastern neighbourhood of São Paulo. From Phoebe and Madalena's comments we can also derive that access is not only shaped by large-scale structures and processes like built environments, economic developments or government investment in physical infrastructures for cycling and walking. The often small-scale actions in terms of how many persons' access can be affected and the time-limited nature of opportunities such as walking groups or cycle training and maintenance sessions suggest a level of fluidity and socio-tempo-spatial differentiation in access that is easily abstracted in research on inequalities in mobility and wellbeing.

> The idea is to encourage the wheelchair user to leave their home and have a more active life. I don't usually donate food staples, I don't usually donate money; I want to encourage people to leave their homes. So, if the guy

says 'I have a wheelchair but it's really bad and I haven't been able to get around', I'll look around for a better wheelchair to give them. The objective is always for them to have a more active life. (Lucas, leader of an organisation that helps disabled people with assistive mobility devices, information provision and group trips, São Paulo)

The diverse nature of the initiatives supporting walking and cycling in São Paulo and London we studied is reinforced by organisations in both cities that help people with disabilities become more mobile. Lucas leads an organisation in São Paulo that runs a range of initiatives, including the provision to those in need of functional wheelchairs and other assistive mobility devices obtained from donors. It is evident that practices such as these can have a major impact on disabled people's access and that a more active life can have many health, social and psychological benefits. The objective of a more active life is also promoted by numerous organisations, including the World Health Organization (WHO) (e.g. WHO, 2015). There is nonetheless an element of ambiguity: while helping to co-constitute a time-space of capability, reinforcing the global norm that people should lead active lives, the initiative also marginalises other ways of being for disabled people which are configured around staying within the home and may be desired by some. Perhaps inevitably, and despite the best of intentions, initiatives and the time-spaces of capability they help to generate can and will also produce their own exclusions.

The excerpt from the interview with Lucas illustrates another point that was also evident from other interviews. Access as defined by Kaufmanm and colleagues cannot be equated to a capability. More is required to turn the opportunities, which could be interpreted as what geographers, transport researchers and urban planners call accessibility, into a capability. This is where competencies play an important role.

Competencies
Among the initiatives supporting walking and cycling in São Paulo that we engaged with during the empirical research, the cultivation of skills and abilities was a key concern and objective. Many concentrated, predictably, on the operational and kinaesthetic skills of how to cycle or walk safely and competently and on the navigational skills of how to get to places while avoiding interpersonal and traffic-related dangers. The former and the latter are exemplified by the initiatives in which Phoebe and Lucas were involved, respectively. Even the walking group

in which Madalena participated cultivated operational and navigational skills and abilities, although this was not an explicit objective. All cases discussed above foreground the collective character of how skills and abilities develop, that is, how interactions between people, technological artefacts, material landscapes, discourse, atmospheres and so forth coalesce into skills and abilities that come to reside in individual body-minds.

Nonetheless, the conditions for the development and sedimentation of such skills and abilities need to be perceived and experienced as somehow right. And many of the initiatives in our research dedicated extensive efforts to the creation of those conditions, seeking to produce time-spaces that are at once secure, socially integrative, capability cultivating and even therapeutic. These points are perhaps best demonstrated through an initiative housed in a somewhat rundown space below an apartment block in London where bicycle maintenance and repair are taught to, and learnt by, cis-gendered women and gender-variant individuals. Bicycle maintenance and repair skills and abilities are very often overlooked in mainstream policy attempts to encourage cycling but nonetheless are of critical importance to longer-term uptake of this form of mobility, and therefore another key concern for many initiatives in our study.

Interviewees from those initiatives highlighted that bicycle breakdown, sometimes as easily fixable as a punctured tyre, was a key moment when poor and otherwise disadvantaged individuals abandon bicycle use and thus become more transport-disadvantaged than they frequently already were when still cycling. The monetary costs of professional maintenance and repair were a major factor in this, as was – particularly in areas further away from the city centre in São Paulo – the low accessibility to such services. For cis-women and gender-variant individuals, the hegemonic masculinities in bicycle maintenance and repair facilities can constitute extra challenges, often triggering feelings of being ill at ease. In fact, it was exactly such feelings that led to the emergence of the aforementioned London initiative for cis-women and gender-variant people, as its initiator explained when interviewed:

> I went in with the idea that I wanted to do [name of a cycling initiative in London] so I needed to get skills. And whilst doing the course, I felt so, like, uncomfortable by how my tutor made me feel. And I was just generally made to feel in that environment as a woman I think, and it was

to do with being a woman ... But it just made me even more clear that when I met Mary, and I said to [her], 'Oh God, I'm just having a really hard time doing my course.' Mary knew exactly which place and why ... although it was hard, it was also really good because I think it made us both like, 'okay, this is how we want to create a space ...' (Linda, initiator of an initiative providing bicycle maintenance and repair instruction to women and gender-variant people, London)

The cultivation of bicycle maintenance and repair skills and abilities as a distinct set of functionings and capabilities not only resulted in the fixing of bicycles already owned or used by workshop or session participants; it also made donated or otherwise acquired old bicycles fit for use by people who previously had no access to bicycles. This, for instance, is what another London initiative that specifically targets refugees and asylum seekers does. One of its staff members, Susan, also highlighted how social integration, security, restoration and capability building are closely interwoven, and she added the hedonic element of pleasure ('fun') – missing from the heuristic classification of time-spaces of wellbeing outlined earlier – to the mix. It is the entanglement of those qualities of the initiative's time-spaces that generates belonging, commitment and a more durable community. The concept of assemblage (Deleuze and Guattari, 1987) is particularly useful in this context because it draws attention, firstly, to how a constantly changing set of elements comes together and collectively generates new elements with a character and qualities that cannot be understood without reference to the process of coming together and interaction from which they have emerged. Secondly, the assemblage concept also highlights how what is generated across different moments (workshops, days, etc.) in the space of the initiative is never quite the same and is always multiple. Bicycle maintenance and repair functionings and capabilities are but one outcome and not necessarily the most important one. The wellbeing generated through the initiative Susan is involved in is complex, and even highlighting the close connections between capabilities, practices and experiences may not capture that complexity adequately.

> Lots of people are new to the area, and they're looking at a way to integrate with the community and build a new skill set ... there are a lot of people who have got bikes from us who come back to improve their maintenance skills, to maintain their own bikes, to help get other people cycling as well. And I think a lot of that coming back, it's not just about the bikes, it's about there being a bit of a community and everybody just doing stuff together

and, you know, not actually coming because we were a refugee service centre and we're providing this that and the other, but it's just like, you know, you come to do something that's quite fun and hanging out with people who are all on the same page and being treated like a human being. (Susan, staff member of an organisation offering various cycling-related activities to refugees and asylum seekers, London)

Appropriation

Competencies go a long way in turning the possibilities referred to as access by Kaufmann and colleagues into capabilities as 'real freedoms or opportunities to achieve functionings' (Robeyns, 2017: 39). Yet our empirical material suggests that certain dispositions are also required for the capability to cycle or walk. In practice, the motility constituents of competencies and appropriation may be difficult to separate; however, if the aim is to understand how the capability to walk or cycle is generated in situations of disadvantage in unequal cities, there is some analytical usefulness to the separation. Consider Marcos, initiator of an organisation that takes people – mostly middle-aged women – for walks through difficult neighbourhoods in peripheral São Paulo.

> The news programmes in [the all-news radio network], the killing, you get scared of leaving your home. It isn't like that, right. The more you occupy the streets, the less violence you'll have and more people you will have on the streets. If the person stays at home, it's because she is afraid, and the street is left empty and you might have muggings and stuff. I've been for a jog to the neighbourhood called Cidade Tiradentes that everyone is afraid of. Also we had a good group walking there. And it wasn't all that, we went there, jogged and came back, no worries. People said: 'wow, aren't you afraid?' It looks like you would be mugged just by going there. And this has nothing to do with reality, right. (Marcos, leader of a walking group initiative in peripheral neighbourhoods, São Paulo)

His words can be interpreted to suggest that, over and above access and competencies, a critical disposition towards discourses that instil fear of crime and withdrawal from streets as public spaces is key to the generation of the capability to walk and cycle in areas like Cidade Tiradentes – an eastern district of São Paulo developed mostly in the 1980s with some 220,000 inhabitants, more than a quarter of whom live in favelas, and with high levels of poverty, illiteracy and (fear of) crime. Jane Jacobs's (1961) famous ideas about eyes on the street and safety in numbers may well have played a role in shaping his thinking.

His words furthermore suggest that practices as a type of functioning are key to the emergence of such a disposition, which is why the initiative he is leading organises walking groups for local residents. However, as with Lucas's initiatives for disabled people discussed above, there is a certain ambiguity and risk of marginalisation of certain ways of being for individuals. A rational human subject who is inclined to adjust their perceptions and preferences once exposed to the accurate information seems to be presumed in the quotation above. There is, however, ample evidence from diverse social science literatures that preferences are not so easily adapted, nor is fear of crime so easily overcome as the excerpt implies (Koskela and Pain, 2000). Group walks can play an important role in the cultivation of certain dispositions – as Madalena's words above and Jessica's below indeed suggest – but those walks are unlikely to be a sufficient condition alone for those dispositions to emerge more broadly.

Jessica is a regular participant in group walks and bicycle rides in north London. Her words help us better understand when the dispositions that help walking become a capability. Familiarity resulting from repeated exposure ('These walks'), positive eudaimonic and hedonic experience ('confidence', 'being like a bird', 'freedom' and 'It's fabulous') and learning how to navigate and what to keep an eye on from the 'guys' who lead the group walks are all important and seem to have generated in Jessica an ethos of controlled experimentation: a willingness to venture out on her own and be exposed to people and events within a delimited area she knows how to navigate and for which she has a reasonable idea about what to expect. This suggests again that appropriation and competencies as well as their respective roles in capability cultivation are difficult to separate in practice.

> Familiarity makes it a bit easier to walk in an area as it does for cycling ... I feel much better on my own cycling ... These walks do it and the bicycles do it, give you the confidence. I never ever went up to [a particular park] until the guys took me. And once they took me, it's like being a bird [laughs], the freedom of going out there on one's own. It's fabulous ... The guys have told me what to look out for. 'Go this way. Beware that.' (Jessica, participant in group walks and bicycle rides organised by a walking and cycling promotion organisation, London)

It is important not to think of dispositions that are favourable to walking and cycling as static once they have emerged. Just as they are cultivated and generated in particular events, they can also be diminished or transformed in later events, including unpleasant, unforeseen encounters that make the shortcomings of one's skills and abilities for handling certain situations visible and/or induce experiences of pain or dependency. Nevertheless, our interviews also suggest that the functionings made possible through the capabilities generated, in part, from new dispositions triggered the emergence of new competencies, travel horizons, aspirations, expectations and needs. The evolution of appropriation was discussed with great clarity by Antonio, who co-leads an organisation that runs multiple initiatives to support cycling in disadvantaged neighbourhoods, including bicycle maintenance and mechanics workshops, cycling-in-traffic skill lessons, bicycle art festivals and coffee provision at cycling events:

> So, now we have some important [information] that [participants] gave to us, that what they learned changed their lives. Like, many of them start to go to school, to go to a park by bicycle, and to work, to save money from the bus tickets. And also a mother of one of the teenagers, we had a parents' meeting, and they told us, 'Oh, my boy had a interview, a job interview in downtown, and he knows how to get there. I was really impressed because he'd never been there at all.' 'I went riding a bicycle today.' 'Oh from Capão Redondo! Riding a bicycle?' … So they get to know distances and the city better. Because in the beginning, they [didn't] even have the knowledge to dream, so when we ask them, 'Where in the city do you want to go?' Sometimes, they don't know how to say because they only know the neighbourhood and … the nearby park. And then when they get to know downtown, other areas, to see, 'Oh, Paulista Avenue has a very beautiful cycle path. Why don't we have this kind of cycle path in our area?' (Antonio, initiator of multiple cycling-supporting initiatives in disadvantaged neighbourhoods, São Paulo)

According to evaluations of the initiatives' activities, participants' lives had been changed. The increased mobility – the set of capabilities produced by the coming together of access, competencies and appropriation – had opened up all kinds of non-mobility functionings and capabilities, which in turn triggered new competencies (going somewhere 'he'd never been … at all', the 'knowledge to dream') and appropriations such as a desire for a central-city-style network of bicycle lanes that are clearly marked with red paint and bicycle paths that are segregated from pedestrian and vehicular traffic and also marked with red paint.

Propositions

On the basis of the analysis in this chapter, we offer three sets of propositions, a term that conveys their tentativeness and the need for further critical interrogation better than 'conclusions' would do. First, in research focusing on wellbeing among disadvantaged individuals or social groups in deeply unequal cities, a focus on either experiences – be they hedonic, eudaimonic or a combination of both – or capabilities seems to be too narrow and reductive. Thinking about experiences, practices and capabilities as 'entwined becomings' appears to be a more useful point of departure for conceptualisation, thinking about research methodology, and empirical research. The notion of entwined becoming also brings out that wellbeing is never simply a state but is constantly happening and in-the-making. It is continually shaped and reshaped by events involving, and stemming from, assemblages of heterogeneous elements, human and otherwise. Wellbeing is therefore not simply individual but distributed (although this term is perhaps too static to convey ongoing happening), emergent from more-than-individual assemblages and at most articulated in an individualised manner in particular body-minds.

Secondly, while we believe that the kind of liberal interpretation and reworking of Sen's CA proposed in this chapter has considerable potential, various issues merit further attention. One such issue is the distinction between capability and functioning. For Robeyns (2017: 39), '[t]he distinction between functionings and capabilities is between the realised and the effectively possible, in other words, between achievements, on the one hand, and freedoms or opportunities from which one can choose, on the other.' Apart from the question of whether choice is the (main) way through which opportunities are converted into functionings, the distinction between what is realised and what could effectively be realised becomes increasingly blurred when empirical materials are used to identify capabilities. For the case of mobility, Kaufmann's concept of motility is useful in the identification of capabilities. However, once competencies and appropriation are probed empirically using a relational and process-based perspective (albeit in this chapter with empirical material focusing on people whose real freedoms in everyday mobility are quite limited), then the answer to the question 'of whether the person could travel [by bicycle or on foot] if she wanted to' (Robeyns, 2017: 39) comes to resemble what she actually did very closely. Future research should problematise and explore further what formulations like 'effectively possible' and 'real opportunity' actually mean in relation to the capabilities concept.

Finally, the chapter demonstrates that the citizen-led initiatives supporting cycling and walking in São Paulo and London that we have studied can make a difference to the wellbeing of poor and otherwise disadvantaged individuals and groups. They fill gaps left by state and market in the cultivation of certain capabilities, experiences and practices in relation to walking and cycling for individuals and groups who can benefit in many ways from such cultivation. The benefits are not unqualified, however. The limited resources – finance, staff and volunteers, etcetera – and the challenge of reproducing the socially integrative, secure, restorative and otherwise supportive time-spaces that the initiatives co-constitute restrict the number of people who can participate in, and benefit from, the initiatives. Moreover, as with almost any attempt to create an inclusive and intimate environment, the empirical materials discussed above suggests that some marginalisation and even exclusion of certain functionings that are easy to justify from a moral perspective is still occurring. While this implies that the wellbeing benefits of the initiatives studied in this chapter should not be romanticised, it is also clear that they create unique desirable effects that extend beyond the realm of everyday mobility for disadvantaged people in unequal cities in which opportunities to develop capabilities are distributed very unevenly.

Acknowledgements

The research on which this chapter draws is part of the DEPICT (*DE*signing and *P*olicy *I*mplementation for encouraging *C*ycling and walking *T*rips) project, funded by the Economic and Social Research Council (ESRC) (grant ES/N011538/1).

Note

1 Although this interview was conducted primarily in English, the right to come and go, known as *direito de ir e vir* in Portuguese, is a constitutional right in Brazil (art. 5, subsection 15, of the 1988 Federal Constitution). The Portuguese expression thus carries semantic gravity.

References

Ahmed, S. (2010). *The promise of happiness*. Durham, NC: Duke University Press.

Atkinson, S.J. (2013). Beyond components of wellbeing: The effects of relational and situated assemblage. *Topoi*, 32: 137–44.

Ballas, D. (2013). What makes a 'happy city'? *Cities*, 32: S39–S50.

Binkley, S. (2014). *Happiness as enterprise: An essay on neoliberal life*. Albany: State University of New York Press.

Birenboim, A. (2018). The influence of urban environments on our subjective momentary experiences. *Environment and Planning B: Urban Analytics and City Science*, 45(5), 915–32.

Clark, D.A. (2005). Sen's capability approach and the many spaces of human well-being. *The Journal of Development Studies*, 41: 1339–68.

Como Anda. (2017). *Mobilidade a pé: Estado da arte do movimento no Brasil*. Como Anda: online.

Deleuze, G., and Guattari, F. (1987). *A thousand plateaus*. Minneapolis: University of Minnesota Press.

De Vos, J., Schwanen, T., Van Acker, V. and Witlox, F. (2013). Travel and subjective well-being: A focus on findings, methods and future research needs. *Transport Reviews*, 33: 421–42.

Diener, E. (2000). Subjective well-being: The science of happiness and a proposal for a national index. *American Psychologist* 55(1): 34–43.

Flamm, M., and Kaufmann, V. (2006). Operationalising the concept of motility: A qualitative study. *Mobilities*, 1: 167–89.

Fleuret, S. and Atkinson, S. (2007). Wellbeing, health and geography: A critical review and research agenda. *New Zealand Geographer*, 63: 106–18.

Hägerstrand, T. (1970). What about people in regional science? *Papers of the Regional Science Association*, 24: 6–21.

Hansen, W.G. (1959). How accessibility shapes land use. *Journal of American Institute of Planners*, 25: 73–6.

Jacobs, J. (1961). *The death and life of great American cities*. New York: Vintage Books.

Kaufmann, V. (2002). *Re-thinking mobility: Contemporary sociology*. London: Routledge.

Kaufmann, V., Bergman, M.M., and Joye, D. (2004). Motility: Mobility as capital. *International Journal of Urban and Regional Research*, 28: 745–56.

Koskela, H., and Pain, R. (2000). Revisiting fear and place: women's fear of attack and the built environment. *Geoforum*, 31: 269–80.

Litman, T. (2007). *Evaluating accessibility for transportation planning*. Victoria Transport Policy Institute: online.

Metz, D. (2015). Peak car in the big city: Reducing London's transport greenhouse gas emissions. *Case Studies on Transport Policy*, 3: 367–71.

Okuliz-Kozaryn, A. (2015). *Happiness and place: Why life is better outside of the city*. New York: Palgrave Macmillan.
Razvadauskas, F. (2017). Income inequality ranking of the world's major cities. MRX Blog, Euromonitor International, https://blog.euromonitor.com/income-inequality-ranking-worlds-major-cities/, (last accessed 1 November 2019).
Robeyns, I. (2017). *Wellbeing, freedom and social justice: The capability approach re-examined*. Cambridge: Open Book Publishers.
Ryan, R., and Deci, E. (2001). On happiness and human potentials: A review of research on hedonic and eudaimonic wellbeing. *Annual Review of Psychology*, 52: 141–66.
Ryff, C., and Singer, B. (2008). Know thyself and become what you are: A eudaimonic approach to psychological well-being. *Journal of Happiness Studies*, 9: 13–39.
Satterthwaite, D. (2007). *The transition to a predominantly urban world and its underpinnings*. London: IEED.
Schwanen, T. (2018). Towards decolonised knowledge about transport. *Palgrave Communications*, 4: 79.
Schwanen, T., and Wang, D. (2014). Well-being, context, and everyday activities in space and time. *Annals of the Association of American Geographers*, 104: 833–54.
Sen, A. (1999). *Development as freedom*. Oxford: Oxford University Press.
Sen, A. (2008). The economics of happiness and capability. In L. Bruni, F. Comim and M. Pugno (Eds) *Capabilities and happiness*, 16–27. Oxford: Oxford University Press.
SINDIPEÇAS and ABIPEÇAS (2017). *Relatório da frota circulante*. São Paulo: Sindicato Nacional da Indústria de Componentes para Veículos Automotores & Associação Brasileira da Indústria de Autopeças.
Smith, T.S.J., and Reid, L. (2018). Which 'being' in wellbeing? Ontology, wellness and the geographies of happiness. *Progress in Human Geography*, 42(6): 807–29.
Thrift, N. (2008). *Non-representational theory: Space, politics, affect*. London: Routledge.
Tinson, A., Ayrton, C., Barker, K., Born, T.B., and Long, O (2017). *London's poverty profile 2017*. Trust for London, www.trustforlondon.org.uk/publications/londons-poverty-profile-2017/ (last accessed 1 November 2019).
Urry, J. (2007). *Mobilities*. Cambridge: Polity.
White, S.C. (2017). Relational wellbeing: Re-centring the politics of happiness, policy and the self. *Policy & Politics*, 45(2): 121–36.
WHO (2015). *WHO global disability action plan 2014–2021: Better health for all people with disability*. Geneva: WHO.

Winters, J., and Li, Y. (2017). Urbanisation, natural amenities and subjective well-being: Evidence from US counties. *Urban Studies*, 54: 1956–73.

Yates, L. (2015). Rethinking prefiguration: Alternatives, micropolitics and goals in social movements. *Social Movement Studies*, 14: 1–21.

5

Urban (sanitation) transformation in China: a Toilet Revolution and its socio-eco-technical entanglements

Deljana Iossifova

Sanitation is entangled with material infrastructure, policy landscapes and everyday practices, encompassing underpinning value, belief and norm systems. In this chapter, I argue that sanitation must be studied as more than an engineered system in order to design targeted interventions towards more sustainable futures. I reflect on the ways in which ideals of the networked city have perpetuated urban governance, planning and design and look at the ways in which they are embedded within China's ongoing Toilet Revolution. I then propose that practice theory, in conjunction with a wider understanding of socio-spatial complexity, has much to offer when we seek to unravel the socio-eco-technical entanglements of sanitation. In line with emerging urban scholarship, I argue that such an approach would help to transcend the traditional dualism of stressing either economic processes or culture, identity and representation when analysing and theorising cities (Sheppard, Leitner and Maringanti, 2013; Leitner and Sheppard, 2016). I conclude that research on the socio-eco-technical co-evolution of sanitation practice and other systems is urgently needed to inform innovative policies, planning and design.

Fantasies of networked cities

The networked city – a city ordered by its infrastructural networks (Dupuy, 2008) – remains the subject of aspiration among policy makers and planners globally and persists in its perception as attainable for any city anywhere. Planning and investment around the world still cater to the ideal of the networked city as a symbol of modernity and progress.

The networked city is conceived as an ensemble, containing (1) networks of infrastructure for the exchange of ideas, waste, power and people; (2) one or more public utility providers; (3) passive consumers as customers; (4) infrastructure provided or regulated by the state; and (5) land use regulated by urban planning and public services available to all (Monstadt and Schramm, 2017; Dupuy, 2008; Monstadt and Schramm, 2013; Coutard and Rutherford, 2015). The theoretical and practical assumptions underpinning the dominance of water-borne systems are embedded in educational systems and perpetuated in the praxis of planning, constructing and inhabiting of modern cities (Richardson, 2012; Berndtsson, 2006; Marks, Martin and Zadoroznyj, 2008). Urban planning, policy and intervention strategies in the water domain reflect aspirations to build a networked city (Monstadt and Schramm, 2017).

In view of the diversity of urban constellations around the world, however, networked cities are an exception rather than the norm (Monstadt and Schramm, 2017). The universal coverage of urban technical networks has been proved infeasible for various reasons: technical networks can cost too much; in most cases, they do not use resources sustainably; and they are hardly ever flexible enough to adapt to rapid urban change, let alone economic or environmental challenges resulting from global crises (Van Vliet, Spaargaren and Oosterveer, 2010).

Existing models of the orderly and networked city and its dependency on singular solutions – such as water-borne sanitation – have long been proved outdated and can, in fact, entrench existing and create new inequality dynamics (McFarlane, Desai and Graham, 2014; Iossifova, 2015). The possible negative implications of water-borne sanitation systems (especially in resource-poor countries) are very well known (e.g., Jewitt, 2011a; Jewitt, 2011b; Black and Fawcett, 2010). It is increasingly recognised that sanitation systems have to be selected in response to the specific context of their implementation (Zurbrügg and Tilley, 2009), and that the development of new technologies must start with the assumption that alternatives to centralised networks may be better suited to conditions in specific contexts (Van Vliet, Spaargaren and Oosterveer, 2010).

Regardless, ideals of the networked city are easily adopted, despite the existence of opportunities for sustainable sanitation transitions, and particularly in countries like China, where the collective memory of more sustainable ways of dealing with human waste is still fresh in people's consciousness and could easily be exploited. Culturally embedded sanitation practices, such as open defecation, were not perceived as problematic until fairly recently. For instance, in India human waste used to be disposed of in private behind bushes and then safely recycled into the soil. This is no longer possible because of rapid population growth, urbanisation and the disappearance of vegetal coverage, leading to open defecation without privacy and with implications for human dignity and health (Ramani, SadreGhazi and Duysters, 2012). Where it is available, the squat toilet – even when connected to a water-borne system – enjoys significantly lower status, which is attributed to the undignified position of its user and the possibility of physical contact with human waste (Srinivas, 2002). Associations of the pit latrine with a 'return' to nature and squalid living conditions contribute to cultural notions of social and economic development that are firmly tied to the flushing toilet (Jewitt, 2011a; Jewitt, 2011b; Jewitt and Ryley, 2014). The flushing toilet itself is today a 'symbol of cultural development and civilisation' and the toilet bowl 'the seat of Western superiority' (Richardson, 2012: 704). It removes human waste from the home in a matter of seconds – 'out of sight, out of mind' (Richardson, 2012).

Urban (sanitation) transformations in China

As is well known, China's recent urban revolution has likely transformed every aspect of everyday life for the country's urban and rural residents (Wang, 2004; Wu, 2007; Campanella, 2008; Ren, 2013). Cities have experienced the displacement of former inner-city residents to the urban fringes (e.g. Shao, 2013); the replacement of former low-income residential areas with new-built gated compounds and commercial districts for a new urban middle class (e.g. He and Liu, 2010); and rural-to-urban migration on an unprecedented scale (e.g., Hussain and Wang, 2010). These processes have contributed to the rise of mounting challenges in relation to the provision of affordable housing, education and, much neglected in the scholarly literature, universal sanitation and the handling of human waste. As rural-to-urban migrants agglomerate in older and impoverished neighbourhoods without access to sanitation in private homes, they have to rely on public toilets as municipalities struggle to develop appropriate responses to their sanitation needs (Iossifova, 2015; Zhou and Zhou, 2018).

In this context, rethinking sanitation – under conditions of rapid urban transformation – seems sensible. The percentage of urban residents forced to defecate in the open in China's cities has been reported to have doubled between 1990 and 2008 (World Health Organization (WHO)/ United Nations Child Agency (UNICEF), 2010). More recent statistics indicate that 86 per cent of urban residents had access to 'at least basic' sanitation in 2015 – up from 77 per cent in 2000 – and that 73 per cent of urban residents accessed 'safely managed' sanitation facilities (WHO/UNICEF, 2017). Yet an estimated 17 million households still did not have access to a private or public 'sanitary toilet' (Cheng et al., 2018).[1] Most adversely affected by exclusion from access to 'modern' sanitation infrastructure are rural-to-urban migrants and the elderly (Iossifova, 2015).

Technically, sanitation is understood as the provision of clean water and the safe removal of human waste. A sanitation system generally encompasses the storage, collection, transport, treatment and discharge or reuse of human waste (Tilley et al., 2008). For instance, while sanitation service networks usually include the steps of 'emptying, collection, transport, storage, treatment (e.g. composting) and utilisation', sewage systems contain fewer steps, namely capture, treatment and disposal (Uddin et al., 2015). Different sanitation systems carry different and wide-ranging implications for the environment on the urban, regional and larger scales, depending on the way in which human waste is treated.

In contemporary China, urban transformation and more recent efforts to 'construct a socialist countryside' (Perry, 2011), among other processes, have produced two main types of coexisting sanitation systems: service-networked sanitation and sewage-based sanitation. Until not too long ago, night soil (faecal sludge) was produced and stored by households, collected by night soil collectors and transported to the countryside, where it was bought by farmers and composted to be used as fertiliser for the production of food – which, in turn, was sold to urban residents (King, 1911; Yu, 2010). Human waste was considered a valuable commodity (Crow, 1937) and treated accordingly in a closed-loop, service-networked sanitation system.

Changing health and hygiene expectations, entangled with efforts of nation-building, motivated a series of campaigns to abandon and replace the traditional night soil collection system over time. For instance, the State Council's Patriotic Health Campaign in the 1950s led to the establishment of health campaign committees at all levels of governance to oversee its implementation (Yang, 2004). When China embarked on its journey to opening up and reforms in the late 1970s, the Patriotic Health Campaign was marginalised, and the focus shifted to rapid economic development. In line with the start of rapid urban redevelopment in the 1980s, a more integrated approach to water supply, toilet retrofitting and health education was introduced (Cheng et al., 2018). The anthropologist Jiaming Zhu's (1988) public call for a 'toilet revolution' (*cesuo geming*) in the late 1980s led to an increase in the discussion of the topic in Chinese media. Rural toilet retrofitting became particularly popular in the 1990s, when the ownership of a 'sanitary toilet' in rural areas jumped from less than 40 to 75 per cent in six years (Hu et al., 2016). In 2014 the National Urban and Rural Environmental Sanitation Clean Action Plan (2015–2020) set a target of 85 per cent for 'sanitary toilet' coverage in rural areas by 2020 (Cheng et al., 2018). Most recently, this target was pushed to 100 per cent as part of the Healthy China 2030 programme (State Council, 2016).

Healthy China 2030 is a new national strategy linked with the country's attempt to rebalance the national economy towards diversification, sustainable levels of growth and more even distribution of benefits, dubbed the 'New Normal' (Hu, 2015). The initiative builds on the four principles of (1) making health a priority; (2) introducing reform and innovation; (3) scientific development (to reduce gaps in basic health services); and (4) fairness and justice, placing the emphasis on rural and remote areas (Tan, Liu and Shao, 2017). Progress is to be measured using thirteen core indicators assessing, among other factors, the health of the environment through the quality of surface water, which is directly related to questions of sanitation (Tan, Liu and Shao, 2017).

Most recently, in April 2015, President Xi called for a renewed Toilet Revolution (Haas, 2017). A main reason was reported as Xi's experience of toilets in the countryside and, more particularly, his concern about the impact of their dire state on the tourism sector (Cheng et al., 2018). The foreign visitor in particular is to be placated, since it is assumed that the 'stench and filth of many Chinese toilets horrifies foreigners' (Haas, 2017). The China National Tourism Administration is said to have planned the upgrading of 25,000 existing public toilets and the construction of 33,500 new ones in tourist areas over three years – with more Western-style toilets yet to be built (Cheng et al., 2018). In an interesting turn, government officials across the country are now being criticised increasingly for wasting money on over-the-top public toilet improvements designed to gain them recognition (and promotion) in Beijing (Kuo, 2018).

Joining in with the ubiquitous propaganda around the Internet of Things, smart electrical appliances, smart buildings and smart cities, toilets are now expected not only to be cleaner than ever before, but also 'smart' ('China plans one last push', 2017). For instance, to aid the sustainable use of toilet paper (and prevent its theft) smart public toilets are known to scan one's face before suspending just about enough paper for a single wipe (Xu, 2018).

The Toilet Revolution is not only linked with the hope to rejuvenate the market and boost tourism, but also with claims to support the Sustainable Development agenda and help to achieve the Sustainable Development Goals (SDGs) (Cheng et al., 2018). However, it promotes the conventional water toilet and its associated superstructure as the holy grail of sanitation (e.g. Hu et al., 2016; 'China plans one last push', 2017; 'Xi "toilet revolution" faces rural challenge', 2017; Cheng et al., 2018; Haas, 2017; Kuo, 2018; Xu, 2018). For instance, Hu et al. (2016: 5) distinguish between toilets that they consider 'acceptable' for 'developed groups' from those that are not. They conclude that 'waterless toilets', whatever their design, are not comparable 'with the conventional water-flush toilets in convenience and comfort'[2] (Hu et al., 2016: 4). Although six types of 'sanitary toilets' (including modern versions of ecological sanitation toilets, such as urine–faeces division toilets) are currently being subsidised by the government, the water-flush toilet continues to be the preferred option among China's urban and rural residents (Hu et al., 2016).

Of course, improved sanitation contributes to preventing disease, reducing the cost of health care and medicine, improving wellbeing and alleviating poverty (Prüss–Ustün et al., 2014; Mills and Cumming, 2016). However, China's transition to water-borne sanitation places the country on a trajectory to become entirely dependent on imported fertiliser for the growth of food crops. The disposal of untreated waste from sewers can result in environmental pollution and degradation with wide-ranging implications for human health and wellbeing (Ju et al., 2005). Treatment does not always form part of the country's waste disposal system, where only less than 48 per cent of the collected urban faecal sludge in 2015 was actually treated (Cheng et al., 2018). China's rapid transition from a closed-loop to the comparatively wasteful sewage-based sanitation system comes at considerable environmental and, ultimately, human cost.

There are explicit tensions between the apparent need to modernise national sanitation infrastructures and the possible implications that such developments may carry for human health, social relations and environmental sustainability. In China, rural-to-urban migrants have limited access to affordable housing and have to depend on low-income neighbourhoods and urban villages for accommodation. Because public toilets are not always available or free to use and central waste collection stations are often demolished first in areas that are selected for redevelopment, migrants frequently have to rely on 'temporary solutions' (such as pit latrines) or simply practice open defecation (Iossifova, 2015). This has implications for everyday health experiences, as well as longer-term health trajectories (Li, 2004; Tong et al., 2011; Liu et al., 2014; Luo and Xie, 2014; Iossifova, 2015).

Another area of concern among policy makers with regard to the provision and management of adequate and inclusive urban sanitation services is the steadily growing and ageing urban population. As a result of economic development, among other factors, the formerly common multi-generation household model is breaking up. As their adult children and grandchildren move to modern residential areas outside city centres, China's urban elderly are left behind in old urban neighbourhoods (Liu et al., 2014). Here, they often lack access to improved sanitation. The younger generations, adopting higher standards of sanitation and hygiene, can be reluctant to visit the elderly, leading to diminishing ties between generations and growing isolation of the sick and elderly (Iossifova, 2015). Sanitation thus carries implications for the everyday lives of an increasing proportion of senior citizens.

To counter the negative effects of purely economic development oriented high-speed urbanisation, China has now put in place its New Type Urbanisation Plan (2014–20). Part of this is the reform of the country's relationship with the environment and its protection (IHEST, 2017). Instead of continuing to expand indefinitely, encroaching on agricultural land and rural livelihoods, the focus of urbanisation and urban transformation is now to be shifted to updating older neighbourhoods and their sanitation systems (Hu and Chen, 2015). However, despite such initiatives, the media tend to argue that poorer urban residents lack morality or the necessary levels of civilisation to participate in urban society, rather than focusing on the assessment of the adequacy of public toilet provision (Zhou and Zhou, 2018). This dominant discourse confirms ideas of superiority among middle- and upper-class urban residents (Zhou and Zhou, 2018; see also Ghertner, 2010, for a discussion of similar phenomena in Delhi, India).

(Towards) a practice approach to sanitation in China and elsewhere

The paragraphs above outline the entanglement of sanitation with material infrastructure, policy landscapes and everyday practices, encompassing underpinning value, belief and norm systems. They help to sketch an argument for the need to study and intervene in sanitation as more than an engineered system in order to design targeted interventions towards more sustainable futures.

This is hardly a new proposition, and a range of different fields have examined water and sanitation as sociotechnical or socio-ecological, as physical or service-networked systems (e.g. Tilley et al., 2008), through the lens of urban political ecology (e.g. Heynen, Kaika and Swyngedouw, 2006; Kaika, 2005), science and technology studies (e.g. Van Vliet, Spaargaren and Oosterveer, 2010), actor-network theory (ANT; e.g. Teh, 2011; Dombroski, 2015) or what has recently been termed 'the infrastructural turn in urban studies' (Coutard and Rutherford, 2015).

The sociotechnical approach, confined to humans and technology, studies the development and use of technology as determined by and shaping social processes and practices over longer periods (Russell and Williams, 2002). ANT is interested in the contribution of the material world to the cultural and political bias of humans and the ways in which they know (Law, 2004; Latour, 2005). ANT can reveal how networks and relations between human and non-human actors change, focusing, in the case of sanitation, on the interaction between people, human excreta, water, toilet bowls, pipes, water bodies and so on (Teh, 2015). In the majority of cases, studies in these fields focus on global north experiences of sociotechnical change and transition. Studies of sanitation infrastructures as sociotechnical assemblages of material configurations, social systems and socio-material practices in the global south are largely interested in the social aspects of sanitation and place these at the centre of their analysis (McFarlane, 2010; McFarlane, Desai and Graham, 2014; McFarlane and Silver, 2017). Theoretical interventions, naturally, are often abstracted to a degree where their relevance and applicability to really existing challenges become questionable, at best. Rather than progressing transdisciplinary work, critical studies are often preoccupied with the agency of marginalised groups and 'the political' (or 'poolitical', as proposed in an awkward double entendre by McFarlane and Silver, 2017).

However, beyond questions of 'metabolic inequality' (e.g. McFarlane, 2013), of social, spatial or otherwise defined justice, sanitation poses key challenges with regard to sustainable development and the wellbeing and health of current and future generations. This is not to dismiss the importance and central role of 'the political' (Mouffe, 2005). Rather, I argue that critical scholarship must find ways to engage with, report on and suggest solutions to theoretical *and* practical questions in order to become and remain relevant beyond its limited academe confines.

Interventions must contribute beyond the development of theory for the sake of theory. They must acknowledge the knowledge needs of practitioners in governance, planning, engineering and design, among many others. At the heart of any approach to sanitation should therefore be the co-creation of transdisciplinary research frameworks (Lang et al., 2012) and the integration of 'current knowledge of how ecology, economics, psychology and sociology collectively contribute to establishing and measuring sustainable wellbeing' (Costanza et al., 2014: 285). Sustainable wellbeing is here understood as the ultimate and overarching aim of sustainable development (Costanza et al., 2016).

Bai et al. (2016) rightly propose that theoretical and practical interventions must be developed from a position of deep knowledge of the social, economic, ecological and political context; they must engage an exploration of desired future visions by a full range of stakeholders through co-design and co-production to increase buy-in on shared goals; they must develop a set of goals with clear objectives and priorities; they must draw in actors from across all sectors (including the public, the private, the community and households); they must recognise the diversity of stakeholders and the complexity of feedback mechanisms (a desirable outcome for some could have negative implications for others); and finally, they must take into account that solutions can never be fixed, but must be flexible and adaptable to respond to new challenges – and new knowledge.

In this sense, I am sympathetic to recent calls for 'provincialising' urban scholarship when analysing and theorising cities (Sheppard, Leitner and Maringanti, 2013; Leitner and Sheppard, 2016) – in other words, progressing an approach which transcends the traditional dualism of stressing either capitalist-economic processes or culture, identity and representation. Sanitation is shaped by and shapes culture, identity and representation; equally, it is interlinked with economic processes across a multitude of scales. A division, therefore, between the mainstream and critical study of urban sanitation is neither necessary nor helpful in times of mounting ecological, economic and political challenges. Scholarship must move beyond the much-emphasised divide between mainstream global urbanism of the kind that seeks to identify 'best practices' for urban governance and builds on ideas of urban infrastructure provision, micro-finance and other mechanisms thought to enable prosperity (liaising with the usual suspects, i.e. the World Bank, the United Nations and other multinational agencies) and the type of 'critical' scholarship with a shared interest in the 'Southern turn' of urbanisation and predominant interest in the exposure of capitalism as the root of all problems (e.g. Roy and Ong, 2011; Edensor and Jayne, 2011; Brenner, 2014).

A systems approach drawing on complexity theory (Bai et al., 2016) is a plausible starting point for the provincialised study of sanitation and its socio-eco-technical entanglements (with 'eco' here referring to both ecological and economic characteristics and processes). In conjunction with this wider framework and in order to unravel how it contains, is shaped by, shapes and is part of ecosystems of critical resources, institutions, cycles and order[3] – that is, human ecosystems 'of biophysical and social factors capable of adaptation and sustainability over time' (Machlis, Force and Burch, 1997: 351) – it makes sense for a social sciences perspective to place the focus on the human practice of sanitation.

Human practice is here initially defined as 'a routinised type of behaviour which consists of several elements, interconnected to one other: forms of bodily activities, forms of mental activities, "things" and their use, a background knowledge in the form of understanding, know-how, states of emotion and motivational knowledge' (Reckwitz, 2002: 249). The human body and how it operates across the various domains entangled with its sustainable functioning are central to such an enquiry. Critical social science often applies a Foucauldian lens that overemphasises the body as an instrument rather than an agent (Wilhite, 2012), subsequently neglecting to report on bodily experiences and their consequences 'in a thorough and convincing manner' (Warde, 2014: 294; see also Oakley, 2016).

There is therefore an urgent need to examine the role of the body and its complex interactions with materials, things, resources, conventions, meanings, space, time and much more. In that these actors continuously interact and co-evolve, they bring about uncertainty and effects across multiple dimensions. Practice theory and, in particular, Shove's notion of 'practice systems … that co-evolve together' (Shove, 2003b: 397), offer a useful conceptual, methodological and analytical apparatus which allows us to place equal weight on and shift the focus across different actors and their interactions.

The practice approach developed from the work of authors who focused on practices in order to understand how households (predominantly in the global north) consume resources in light of current environmental challenges (Miettinen, Samra-Fredericks and Yanow, 2009; Stern, 2003). This work emphasises the changing conventions of comfort, cleanliness and convenience and how they are linked with increasingly intensive resource consumption (Shove, 2003a; Shove, 2003b). For instance, Shove (2003b) notes that the universalisation of indoor comfort conditions has led to intensive resource use in buildings designed to make this experience similar in vastly different geographic, climatic and cultural contexts. As mentioned in the section above, similar processes have taken place in the realm of sanitation and continue to do so, with the rise of the Western-style flush toilet a prime example.

Although changes in 'individual behaviour, daily routines and perhaps even social norms' (Ramani, SadreGhazi and Duysters, 2012: 677) are necessary for any sustainable transition, such changes can also lead to essentially unsustainable practices. Having a shower every day, wearing clean clothing or eating imported food as a result of shifting social norms and 'notions of what it is to be a normal and acceptable member of society' (Shove, 2004: 77) are mundane practices with enormous implications for wider social, economic and environmental systems. Transitioning to substantially more resource-intensive sanitation practices, as in the case of China's Toilet Revolution outlined above, may lead to social exclusion, economic stratification and ecological degradation on unimaginable scales.

Conceptualised in this way, practice analysis allows us to account for structure and agency simultaneously (Warde, 2005) as well as to understand how structures are reproduced and/or transformed through actions (Miettinen, Samra-Fredericks and Yanow, 2009). For instance, from a practice perspective, dominant institutional projects can be conceptualised as 'complex amalgams of past trajectories and current aims and aspirations, many of which are materially sustained and reinforced by the state [including] conventions of family life, systems of provision and consumption, economic relations and more' (Shove, 2014: 425). The state is here inscribed in the reproduction of institutions and systems; it contributes to the reproduction of 'normal and acceptable ways of life' and the patterns of resource consumption associated with them (Shove, 2014: 425). Understanding the links between the emergence, disappearance and circulation of practices and the material elements that are part of practice systems can therefore enable the design of interventions that reconfigure 'the elements of practice; relation between practices; and patterns of recruitment and defecation' of those who practise them (Shove, 2014: 419).

In summary, the notion of practice enables a more comprehensive understanding of how the everyday is located within wider (and narrower) systems, transcending body–mind or socio–material dualisms in the context of research on sanitation. In its engagement with resource use and energy consumption, the practice approach can provide insights that are relevant to sustainability policy and sustainability outcomes (Hand, Shove and Southerton, 2005; Warde, 2005, 2014). Shove (2014: 418) goes as far as to argue that the emergence, persistence and disappearance of practices, as 'recognisable entities that exist across time and space, that depend on inherently provisional integrations of elements, and that are enacted by cohorts of more or less consistent or faithful carriers' (i.e. practitioners), should be at the heart of any policy-oriented research. They should certainly be at the heart of any work on sanitation.

Conclusion

The theoretical and practical assumptions embedded in the study, design, planning, implementation and use of 'sanitation' underpin the dominance of water-borne systems across the world, and they are an important factor in China's current experience. In this chapter, I have reflected on the role of sanitation in China's urban transformation and how the recently announced Toilet Revolution is linked with largely unsustainable ideas of progress. Famously, over thousands of years China operated a largely closed-loop sanitation system which saw the removal of human waste from the city and its reuse as fertiliser for the growth of food in the countryside. A series of campaigns in modern times, motivated by changing conceptions of health and hygiene, led to the gradual dismantlement of this system in favour of increasingly centralised and physically networked urban sanitation infrastructures. The last couple of decades, in particular, have been marked by the rapid expansion of sewage networks in line with high-speed urbanisation. The most recent initiative, President Xi's Toilet Revolution, targets the expansion of public toilet coverage and, in particular, the transformation of sanitation in the countryside. It is designed as a new driver for economic growth and linked with strategies for the development of the country's tourism industry. China is now well on the way to complete the transition from largely closed-loop, service-based sanitation to resource-intensive sewage-based sanitation across urban and rural settings. This threatens to pollute water bodies and, ultimately, adversely affect human health and wellbeing.

Initiatives like China's Toilet Revolution can be exposed as ideologically motivated by misguided conceptions of the networked city and its civilised citizen as well as politically motivated by the promise of economic development and continued approval of existing political conditions. The implications of rapid sanitation transitions for human health, social relations and environmental sustainability are largely unclear. For instance, health outcomes are likely to be detrimental for rural-to-urban migrants in Chinese cities as their needs are not regarded as a priority in terms of sanitation provision. As well as other groups, especially the rapidly growing and ageing population, they are likely to suffer social exclusion, marginalisation and isolation as a result of the lack of access to 'modern' sanitation. Finally, pollution as a result of incomplete or inappropriately implemented sewage systems and the unsustainably intensive use of water – particularly where it is already a scarce resource, for instance in China's western regions – will bring about challenges for the environment. In light of these challenges, research is urgently needed to inform policy and praxis across all levels of governance, planning and implementation.

I argue that theoretical and practical assumptions in relation to sanitation must be challenged from the ground up in order to develop a rich understanding of sanitation needs, challenges and the possibility for future alternatives to standard sanitation interventions. I am sympathetic to recent calls for a provincialised urban scholarship which seeks to transcend the divide between mainstream urbanism (with the progress of strategies for economic development in mind) and 'critical' urban scholarship concerned with the capitalist mode of planetary urbanisation and/or overly sensitive to socio-political aspects. In the context of mounting ecological, economic and political crises, a unified approach to the study of sanitation which takes into account culture, identity and representation as well as predominant economic and ecological processes across a multitude of scales is needed. I suggest that a systems approach drawing on complexity theory and practice theory is a plausible starting point for the unravelling of sanitation and its socio-eco-technical entanglements. The notion of practice enables a more comprehensive understanding of sanitation as located within wider (and narrower) systems, transcending body–mind or socio–material dualisms. Practice analysis accounts simultaneously for structure and agency across time and space. A systems approach combining the analysis of socio-ecological and sociotechnical processes is necessary to capture the complexity of urban sanitation in any context, but particularly where different sanitation systems coexist, interact and coevolve.

Acknowledgements

I would like to thank Dr Alison Browne and Cecilia Alda-Vidal as well as my partners on the Economic and Social Research Council (ESRC) Strategic Network Data and Cities as Complex Adaptive Systems (DACAS) and colleagues at the Urban Studies Institute (University of Antwerp), Cosmopolis (Vrije Universiteit Brussels) and Manchester Architecture Research Group (University of Manchester) for their thoughtful comments and suggestions on the development of this chapter and the larger project of which this is part.

Notes

1 In addition to the 'conventional' water-flushing toilet, the notion of 'sanitary toilet' in China comprises roughly dual-pit alternating, urine–faeces division, biogas-linked and dual-urn toilets (Hu et al., 2016; Cheng et al., 2018). These last three types of toilet fall under the category of ecological sanitation (ecosan), which seeks to prevent pollution, sanitise human interaction with faeces and urine, and recover nutrients for food production in using treated human excreta as an agricultural resource (Haq and Cambridge, 2012; Langergraber and Muellegger, 2005).

2 An often-cited example of unsuccessful ecological sanitation in China is the installation and failure of such a system in the northern city of Erdos. This was installed as a system of urine-diversion dry toilets, low-flush urinals, faeces collection bins, urine tanks, a grey water treatment plant and a composting plant. Despite impeccable implementation, the project failed because of the 'people's desire of good sanitation conditions' (Hu et al., 2016: 13–14). However, Gao (2011) describes how residents poured water and grey water into the urine-diverting toilets because they were not familiar with the system and relied on traditional knowledge. The project was implemented in a way that did not include or allow residents to adapt to eco-san. Eventually, the dry toilets had to be removed and replaced by conventional water-flushed toilets.
3 The human ecosystem framework (Machlis, Force and Burch 1997) combines the study of relationships between (1) resource systems (*ecosystem resources*, such as energy, water, nutrients, material and soil; *cultural resources*, such as organisations, beliefs and myths; and *socio-economic resources*, such as information, labour and capital) and (2) human social systems (*social institutions*, such as health, justice, education, leisure and governance; *social cycles* across different scales (physical, individual, environmental, organisational, etc.); and *systems of social order*, including identity (age, gender, class), norms (formal, informal) and hierarchies (wealth, power, status, knowledge, territory)). The framework has been successfully applied to the study of the social dimensions of ecological change and of the ecological dimensions of social change (e.g. Redman, Grove and Kuby, 2004; Elmqvist et al., 2013).

References

Bai, X., Surveyer, A., Elmqvist, T., Gatzweiler, F.W., Güneralp, B., Parnell, S., Prieur-Richard, A., Shrivastava, P., Siri, J.G., Stafford-Smith, M., Toussaint, J., and Webb, R. (2016). Defining and advancing a systems approach for sustainable cities. *Current Opinion in Environmental Sustainability*, 23: 69–78.

Berndtsson, J.C. (2006). Experiences from the implementation of a urine separation system: Goals, planning, reality. *Building and environment*, 41(4): 427–37.

Black, M., and Fawcett, B. (2010). *The last taboo: Opening the door on the global sanitation crisis*. London: Routledge.

Brenner, N. (ed.) (2014). *Implosions/explosions: Towards a study of planetary urbanization*. Berlin: Jovis.

Campanella, T.J. (2008). *The concrete dragon: China's urban revolution and what it means for the world*. New York: Princeton Architectural Press.

Cheng, S., Li, Z., Nazim Uddin, S.M., Mang, H., Zhou, X., Zhang, J., Zheng, L., and Zhang, L. (2018). Toilet revolution in China. *Journal of Environmental Management*, 216: 347–56.

China plans one last push in the toilet revolution (2017). *The Economist*, 7 December.
Costanza, R., Kubiszewski, I., Giovannini, E., Lovins, H., McGlade, J., Pickett, K.E., Vala Ragnarsdóttir, K., Roberts, D., De Vogli R., and Wilkinson, R. (2014). Time to leave GDP behind. *Nature*, 505(7483): 283–5.
Costanza, R., Daly, L., Fioramonti, L., Giovannini, E., Kubiszewski, I., Mortensen, L.F., Pickett, K.E., Vala Ragnarsdottir, K., De Vogli, R., and Wilkinson, R. (2016). Modelling and measuring sustainable wellbeing in connection with the UN Sustainable Development Goals. *Ecological Economics*, 130: 350–5.
Coutard, O. and Rutherford, J. (2015). *Beyond the networked city: Infrastructure reconfigurations and urban change in the North and South*. London and New York: Routledge.
Crow, C. (1937). *The Chinese are like that*. New York and London: Harper & Brothers.
Dombroski, K. (2015) Multiplying Possibilities: A postdevelopment approach to hygiene and sanitation in Northwest China. *Asia Pacific Viewpoint*, 56, 321–334.
Dupuy, G. (2008). *Urban networks – Network urbanism*. Amsterdam: IT Techne Press.
Edensor, T., and Jayne, M. (eds) (2011). *Urban theory beyond the West: A world of cities*. London and New York: Routledge.
Elmqvist, T., Redman, C.L., Barthel, S., and Costanza, R. (2013). History of urbanization and the missing ecology. In T. Elmqvist, M. Fragkias, J. Goodness, B. Güneralp, P.J. Marcotullio, R.I. McDonald, S. Parnell, M. Schewenius, M. Sendstad, K.C. Seto and C. Wilkinson (eds), *Urbanization, biodiversity and ecosystem services: Challenges and opportunities*, 13–30. Dordrecht: Springer.
Gao, S. (2011). Ecological sanitation in urban China: A case study of the Dongsheng project on applying ecological sanitation in multi-storey buildings. MSc dissertation in Sustainable Development, Temat Institute, Department of Water and Environmental Studies, Linköping University.
Ghertner, D.A. (2010). Calculating without numbers: Aesthetic governmentality in Delhi's slums. *Economy and Society*, 39(2): 185–217.
Haas, B. (2017). Xi Jinping makes China's toilets a number two priority. *The Guardian*, 28 November 2017.
Hand, M., Shove, E., and Southerton, D. (2005). Explaining showering: A discussion of the material, conventional, and temporal dimensions of practice. *Sociological Research Online*, 10(2): 1–13.
Haq, G., and Cambridge, H. (2012). Exploiting the co-benefits of ecological sanitation. *Current Opinion in Environmental Sustainability*, 4(4): 431–5.
He, S., and Liu, Y. (2010). Mechanism and consequences of China's gentrification under market transition. *Scientia Geographica Sinica*, 30(2): 493–502.

Heynen, N.C., Kaika, M., and Swyngedouw, E. (eds) (2006). *In the nature of cities: Urban political ecology and the politics of urban metabolism*. London: Routledge.
Hu, A. (2015). Embracing China's new normal. *Foreign Affairs*, 94 (3): 8–12.
Hu, B., and Chen, C. (2015). New urbanisation under globalisation and the social implications in China. *Asia & the Pacific Policy Studies*, 2(1): 34–43.
Hu, M., Fan, B., Wang, H., Qu, B., and Zhu, S. (2016). Constructing the ecological sanitation: A review on technology and methods. *Journal of Cleaner Production*, 125: 1–21.
Hussain, A., and Wang, Y. (2010). Rural–urban migration in China: Scale, composition, pattern and deprivation. In F. Wu and C. Webster (eds), *Marginalization in urban China: Comparative perspectives*, 133–53. Basingstoke: Palgrave Macmillan.
IHEST (2017). *Urban policies in China*, part 1. Paris: Institut des Hautes Études pour la Science et la Technologie.
Iossifova, D. (2015). Everyday practices of sanitation under uneven urban development in contemporary Shanghai. *Environment and Urbanization*, 27(2): 541–54.
Jewitt, S. (2011a). Geographies of shit: Spatial and temporal variations in attitudes towards human waste. *Progress in Human Geography* 35(5): 608–26.
Jewitt, S. (2011b). Poo gurus? Researching the threats and opportunities presented by human waste. *Applied Geography*, 31(2): 761–9.
Jewitt, S., and Ryley, H. (2014). It's a girl thing: Menstruation, school attendance, spatial mobility and wider gender inequalities in Kenya. *Geoforum*, 56(0): 137–47.
Ju, X., Zhang, F., Bao, X., Römheld, V., and Roelcke, M. (2005). Utilization and management of organic wastes in Chinese agriculture: Past, present and perspectives. *Science in China Series C: Life Sciences* 48(2): 965–79.
Kaika, M. (2005). *City of flows: Modernity, nature, and the city*. New York and London: Routledge.
King, F.H. (1911). *Farmers of forty centuries: or, Permanent agriculture in China, Korea and Japan*. Madison, WI: F.H. King.
Kuo, L. (2018). Japan offers to lend hand in China's 'toilet revolution'. *The Guardian*, 17 April.
Lang, D.J., Wiek, A., Bergmann, M., Stauffacher, M., Martens, P., Moll, P., Swilling, M., and Thomas, C.J. (2012). Transdisciplinary research in sustainability science: Practice, principles, and challenges. *Sustainability Science*, 7(1): 25–43.
Langergraber, G., and Muellegger, E. (2005). Ecological sanitation – A way to solve global sanitation problems? *Environment International*, 31(3): 433–44.
Latour, B. (2005). *Reassembling the social: An introduction to actor-network-theory*. Oxford: Oxford University Press.

Law, J. (2004). *After method: Mess in social science research*. London and New York: Routledge.

Leitner, H., and Sheppard, E. (2016). Provincializing critical urban theory: Extending the ecosystem of possibilities. *International Journal of Urban and Regional Research*, 40(1): 228–35.

Li, B. (2004). Urban social exclusion in transitional China. CASEpaper 82, Centre for Analysis of Social Exclusion, London School of Economics.

Liu, L., Fu, Y., Qu, L., and Wang, Y. (2014). Home health care needs and willingness to pay for home health care among the empty-nest elderly in Shanghai, China. *International Journal of Gerontology*, 8(1): 31–6.

Luo, W., and Xie, Y. (2014). Socio-economic disparities in mortality among the elderly in China. *Population Studies*, 68(3): 305–20.

Machlis, G.E., Force, J.E., and Burch, W.R. (1997). The human ecosystem: Part I: The human ecosystem as an organizing concept in ecosystem management. *Society & Natural Resources: An International Journal*, 10(4): 347–67.

Marks, J., Martin, B., and Zadoroznyj, M. (2008). How Australians order acceptance of recycled water: National baseline data. *Journal of Sociology*, 44(1): 83–99.

McFarlane, C. (2010). Infrastructure, interruption and inequality: Urban life in the global south. In S. Graham (ed.), *Disrupted cities: When infrastructure fails*, 131–44. New York: Routledge.

McFarlane, C. (2013). Metabolic inequalities in Mumbai: Beyond telescopic urbanism. *City*, 17(4): 498–503.

McFarlane, C., Desai, R., and Graham, S. (2014). Informal urban sanitation: Everyday life, poverty, and comparison. *Annals of the Association of American Geographers*, 104(5): 989–1011.

McFarlane, C., and Silver, J. (2017). The poolitical city: 'Seeing sanitation' and making the urban political in Cape Town. *Antipode*, 49 (1): 125–48.

Miettinen, R., Samra-Fredericks, D., and Yanow, D. (2009). Re-turn to practice: An introductory essay. *Organization Studies*, 30(12): 1309–27.

Mills, J.E., and Cumming, O. (2016). The impact of water, sanitation and hygiene on key health and social outcomes: Review of evidence. UNICEF and SHARE, www.unicef.org/wash/files/The_Impact_of_WASH_on_Key_Social_and_Health_Outcomes_Review_of_Evidence.pdf (last accessed 1 November 2015).

Monstadt, J., and Schramm, S. (2013). 'Beyond the networked city? Suburban constellations in water and sanitation systems'. In R. Keil (ed.), *Suburban constellations*, 85–94. Berlin: JOVIS.

Monstadt, J., and Schramm, S. (2017). Toward the networked city? Translating technological ideals and planning models in water and sanitation systems in Dar Es Salaam. *International Journal of Urban and Regional Research*, 41(1): 104–25.

Mouffe, C. (2005). *On the political*. London and New York: Routledge.

Oakley, A. (2016). A small sociology of maternal memory. *The Sociological Review*, 64(3): 533–49.

Perry, E.J. (2011). From mass campaigns to managed campaigns: Constructing a new socialist countryside. In S. Heilmann and E.J. Pery (eds), *Mao's invisible hand: The political foundations of adaptive governance in China*, 30–61. Cambridge, MA: Harvard University Press.

Prüss-Ustün, A., Bartram, J., Clasen, T., Colford, J.M., Cumming, O., Curtis, V., Bonjour, S., Dangour, A.D., De France, J., and Fewtrell, L. (2014). Burden of disease from inadequate water, sanitation and hygiene in low-and middle-income settings: a retrospective analysis of data from 145 countries. *Tropical Medicine & International Health*, 19(8): 894–905.

Ramani, S.V., SadreGhazi, S., and Duysters, G. (2012). On the diffusion of toilets as bottom of the pyramid innovation: Lessons from sanitation entrepreneurs. *Technological Forecasting and Social Change*, 79(4): 676–87.

Reckwitz, A. (2002). Toward a theory of social practices: A development in culturalist theorizing. *European Journal of Social Theory*, 5(2): 243–63.

Redman, C.L., Grove, J.M., and Kuby, L.H. (2004). Integrating social science into the long-term ecological research (LTER) network: Social dimensions of ecological change and ecological dimensions of social change. *Ecosystems*, 7(2): 161–71.

Ren, X. (2013). *Urban China*. Cambridge: Polity Press.

Richardson, A. (2012). A new world ordure? Thoughts on the use of humanure in developed cities. *City*, 16(6): 700–12.

Roy, A., and Ong, A. (eds) (2011). *Worlding cities: Asian experiments and the art of being global*. Chichester: John Wiley & Sons.

Russell, S., and Williams, R. (2002). Social shaping of technology: Frameworks, findings and implications for policy with glossary of social shaping concepts. In H. Sørensen and R. Williams (eds), *Shaping technology, guiding policy: Concepts, spaces and tools*, 37–132. Cheltenham: Edward Elgar.

Shao, Q. (2013). *Shanghai gone: Domicide and defiance in a Chinese megacity*. Lanham, MD: Rowman & Littlefield.

Sheppard, E., Leitner, H., and Maringanti, A. (2013). Provincializing global urbanism: A manifesto. *Urban Geography*, 34(7): 893–900.

Shove, E. (2003a). *Comfort, cleanliness and convenience: The social organization of normality*. London: Berg.

Shove, E. 2003b. Converging conventions of comfort, cleanliness and convenience. *Journal of Consumer Policy*, 26(4): 395–418.

Shove, E. (2004). Sustainability, system innovation and the laundry. In B. Elzen, F.W. Geels and K. Green (eds), *System innovation and the transition to sustainability: Theory, evidence and policy*, 76–94. Cheltenham: Edward Elgar.

Shove, E. (2014). Putting practice into policy: Reconfiguring questions of consumption and climate change. *Contemporary Social Science*, 9(4): 415–29.

Srinivas, T. (2002). Flush with success: Bathing, defecation, worship, and social change in South India. *Space and Culture*, 5(4): 368–86.
State Council (2016). *Healthy China 2030 program planning*. Beijing: State Council.
Stern, D.G. (2003). The practical turn. In S.P. Turner and P.A. Roth (eds), *The Blackwell guide to the philosophy of the social sciences*, 185–206. Malden, MA, and Oxford: Blackwell Publishing Ltd.
Tan, X., Liu, X., and Shao, H. (2017). Healthy China 2030: A vision for health care. *Value in Health Regional Issues*, 12: 112–14.
Teh, T. (2011). Hydro-urbanism: Reconfiguring the urban water-cycle in the lower Lea river basin, London. PhD dissertation in Civil, Environmental and Geomatic Engineering, University College London.
Teh, T. (2015). Bypassing the flush, creating new resources: Analysing alternative sanitation futures in London. *Local Environment*, 20(3): 335–49.
Tilley, E., Ulrich, L., Lüthi, C., Reymond, P., and Zurbrügg, C. (2008). *Compendium of sanitation systems and technologies*. Dübendorf, Switzerland: Swiss Federal Institute of Aquatic Science and Technology (Eawag).
Tong, H., Lai, D.W., Zeng, Q., and Xu, W. (2011). Effects of social exclusion on depressive symptoms: Elderly Chinese living alone in Shanghai, China. *Journal of Cross-Cultural Gerontology*, 26(4): 349–64.
Uddin, S.M.N., Li, Z., Mahmood, I.B., Lapegue, J., Adamowski, J.F., Donati, P.F., Huba, E.M., Mang, H., Avirmed, B., and Cheng, S. (2015). Evaluation of a closed-loop sanitation system in a cold climate: a case from peri-urban areas of Mongolia. *Environment and Urbanization*, 27(2): 455–72.
Van Vliet, B., Spaargaren, G., and Oosterveer, P. (2010). *Social perspectives on the sanitation challenge*. New York: Springer.
Wang, Y.P. (2004). *Urban poverty, housing and social change in China*. London: Routledge.
Warde, A. (2005). Consumption and theories of practice. *Journal of Consumer Culture*, 5(2): 131–53.
Warde, A. (2014). After taste: Culture, consumption and theories of practice. *Journal of Consumer Culture*, 14 (3): 279–303.
WHO/UNICEF (2010). *Progress on sanitation and drinking-water: 2010 update*. Geneva: WHO and UNICEF.
WHO/UNICEF (2017). *Progress on drinking water, sanitation and hygiene: 2017 update and SDG baselines (annexes)*. Geneva: WHO and UNICEF.
Wilhite, H. (2012). Towards a better accounting of the roles of body, things and habits in consumption. In A. Warde and D. Southerton (eds), *COLLeGIUM: Studies across disciplines in the humanities and social sciences*, 87–99. Helsinki: Helsinki Collegium for Advanced Studies.
Wu, F. (2007). *China's emerging cities: The making of new urbanism*. Abingdon: Routledge.

Xi 'Toilet Revolution' faces rural challenge (2017). *South China Morning* Post, 5 December.

Xu, Y. (2018). China's 'Toilet Revolution' is flush with lavish loos. NPR, 3 February, www.npr.org/sections/goatsandsoda/2018/02/03/579283921/chinas-toilet-revolution-is-flush-with-lavish-loos (last accessed 1 November 2019).

Yang, N. (2004). Disease prevention, social mobilization and spatial politics: The anti germ-warfare incident of 1952 and the 'Patriotic Health Campaign'. *The Chinese Historical Review*, 11(2): 155–82.

Yu, X. (2010). The treatment of night soil and waste in modern China. In Q. Liang, A. Ki, C. Leung and C. Furth (eds), *Health and hygiene in Chinese East Asia: Policies and publics in the long twentieth century*, 51–72. Durham, NC: Duke University Press.

Zhou, X., and Zhou, C. (2018). Cesuo geming zai zhongguo de yuanqi, xianzhuang yu yanshuo [The origin, status quo, and expression of 'Toilet Revolution' in China]. *Zhongyuan wenhua yanjiu* [*Central Plains Culture Research*], 2018(1): 22–31.

Zhu, J. (ed.) (1988). *Zhongguo: xuyao cesuo geming* [*China needs a toilet revolution*]. Shanghai: Sanian Shudian Shanghai Fendian.

Zurbrügg, C., and Tilley, E. (2009). A system perspective in sanitation – Human waste from cradle to grave and reincarnation. *Desalination*, 248(1–3): 410–17.

6

The food environment and health in African cities: analysing the linkages and exploring possibilities for improving health and wellbeing

Warren Smit

The 'food environment' of cities can be defined as the location and type of food sources, as well as the broader environmental factors that affect the production, retail and consumption of food in cities (such as levels of infrastructure). The food environment of cities has an impact on the health and wellbeing of residents, although the measurement of this impact has proved to be difficult. Although there is a growing body of research on the effect of food environments on health, this relationship has been under-recognised and under-studied in the global south (Herforth and Ahmed, 2015; Turner et al., 2017).

Understanding the food environments of African cities is important because there are high levels of food insecurity in African cities, driven by high levels of poverty and income variability (Battersby and Watson, 2018), and interventions in urban food environments can potentially contribute to improving health outcomes. Food security can be defined as people's 'physical, social and economic access to sufficient, safe and nutritious food to meet their dietary needs and food preferences for an active and healthy life' (Food and Agriculture Organization of the United Nations (FAO), 2009: 1). The reality in African cities is very different. A survey of food security in eleven southern African cities found 76 per cent of sampled households to be moderately or severely food-insecure, in other words they often do not have enough food to eat for their minimum dietary needs (Frayne et al., 2010). An estimated 47 per cent of residents in Nairobi, Kenya, are estimated to be food-insecure, and food insecurity is highest in slum areas: for example, 85 per cent of residents of slum areas of Nairobi are estimated to be food-insecure (Dixon et al., 2007; Kimani-Murage et al., 2014). Food insecurity is exacerbated by low levels of dietary diversity; food-insecure households in southern Africa typically only eat three to five different food groups, compared with an average of eight for food-secure households (Frayne et al., 2010). These high levels of food insecurity and lack of dietary diversity have an enormous impact on health and wellbeing. For example, surveys in Accra, Ghana, and Kitwe, Zambia, found 'disturbingly high levels of stunting (chronic malnutrition) and wasting (acute malnutrition) among children in both the lowest income and the poor–middle income populations' (de Zeeuw and Prain, 2011). Unhealthy eating patterns have also led towards a 'dual burden' of undernutrition and obesity for poor households, often within the same household (Doak et al., 2004).

This chapter draws on work undertaken as part of a project funded by the Economic and Social Research Council (ESRC), Consuming Urban Poverty, on governing food systems to alleviate poverty in secondary cities in Africa (Kisumu in Kenya, Kitwe in Zambia, and Epworth, part of the Harare city-region in Zimbabwe), as well as other work undertaken by the African Centre for Cities on health, food and urban development in Cape Town (South Africa). The survey findings drawn on in this chapter include workshops and interviews in Cape Town, a food retail survey in Kisumu, and food consumption surveys in Kisumu and in Kitwe.

First, the chapter examines the food environments of African cities, with a focus on the built environment, highlighting the diverse range of food outlets and complex patterns of food access. Kisumu in Kenya is used as an example. Second, the chapter explores the multi-faceted ways in which the food environment of cities can afffect human health and wellbeing. Finally, the chapter discusses possibilities for how food environments that are more conducive to health and wellbeing can be created and sustained, and suggests some avenues for future research on urban food environments.

The concept of urban food environments

Food environments can be defined in various ways. Broadly, building on the socio-ecological perspective, they can be defined as 'the collective physical, economic, policy and sociocultural surroundings, opportunities and conditions that influence people's food and beverage choices and nutritional status' (Swinburn et al., 2013: 25). Food environments are essentially the context in which the acquisition and consumption of food occurs, providing a series of opportunities and constraints that influence decisions about what to eat (FAO, 2016).

Most studies of urban food environments have focused on the categorisation, measurement and geographic analysis of different types of food outlet (McKinnnon et al., 2009). Various tools, such as the Food Environment Classification Tool (Lake et al., 2010), and measurement indices, such as the Retail Food Environment Index (Spence et al., 2009), have been developed. The Retail Food Environment Index is a simple measure of food environments (the number of fast-food outlets divided by the number of supermarkets and grocery stores), based on the questionable assumption that supermarkets and grocery stores always sell healthier food than convenience stores and fast-food outlets.

Glanz et al. (2007) distinguish between three types of food environment: the community nutrition environment (essentially the number, type and location of stores within a defined geographical area), the within-store consumer nutrition environment (availability of healthy options, price, nutrition information) and the organisational nutrition environment (home, school or work). Similarly, one can distinguish between the 'external food environment' (which has an impact on the availability of food) and the 'personal food environment' (which includes factors such as accessibility, affordability, convenience and desirability) (Turner et al., 2017).

The statistically significant findings of a relationship between the physical urban environment and health have been modest. For example, a systematic review of thirty-eight studies 'found moderate evidence in support of the causal hypothesis that neighbourhood food environments influence dietary health' (Caspi et al., 2012: 1181). This is not necessarily because there is not a significant relationship but is perhaps more a reflection of the fact that the overall quality of food environment research has generally been low (Cobb et al., 2015) and because the research was arguably often not focusing on the right questions. For example, Zenk et al. (2005) have noted that although the focus of much food environment research has been on distance to food outlets (which is easy to measure), in fact, travel time instead of distance should be considered, and social barriers (such as crime) and individual mobility issues need to be given more prominence.

Recent research on food environments has highlighted the importance of understanding the multiple environments in which people spend their time on accessing and consuming food (Townshend and Lake, 2017). There is a need to understand 'foodways', which relate to the interplay between individual processes and broader context (Alkon et al., 2013; Cannuscio, Weiss and Asch, 2010). The term 'foodways' refers to 'the cultural and social practices that affect food consumption, including how and what communities eat, where and how they shop and what motivates their food preferences' (Alkon et al., 2013: 127). Alkon et al. (2013: 126) conclude that 'cost, not lack of knowledge or physical distance, is the primary barrier to healthy food access, and that low-income people employ a wide variety of strategies to obtain the foods they prefer at prices they can afford'.

In this chapter, I focus on the built-environment aspects of the 'community' or 'external' food environments of cities: for example, on the location and type of food outlets and food vendors, and the extent of urban agriculture. At a higher level, food environments also include broader contextual factors that influence the production, retail and consumption of food in cities (such as levels of infrastructure and enforcement of regulations related to the built environment).

Urban food environments in African cities

Urban food environments in cities in Africa and elsewhere in the global south are characterised by the 'co-existence of formal and informal food markets, as well as non-market based food sources such as own production and food transfers' (Turner et al., 2017: 3). A survey of southern African cities reflected the complexity of foodways, with the main sources of food including supermarkets, informal markets, small shops, self-production (e.g. growing of vegetables), sharing of food, borrowing of food, food remittances, community food kitchens and food aid (Frayne et al., 2010).

The term 'formal' is usually used to apply to legal or officially registered activities or entities, while the term 'informal' is used to apply to extra-legal or unregistered activities or entities (Hansen and Vaa, 2004). It should be borne in mind that classifying a particular activity or entity as solely formal or informal is usually impossible: there generally are multiple layers of formality and informality. For example, 'informal traders' may be formal in many respects – they may pay for a permit from the local government and may have a health permit – but informal in other respects, in that, for example, they do not pay company or individual income tax, or the physical structure they use does not comply with planning and building regulations. Formality and informality should be regarded as a continuum rather than a dichotomy, and I use the terms to refer to the respective ends of the continuum.

Most food outlets in African cities are at the informal end of the formality–informality continuum, and they account for a large proportion of food sales. For example, the Urban Consumption Survey in Zambia found in 2007–8 that 42 per cent of households primarily bought food from informal retailers. The informal economy was a particularly important source for chicken and poultry (73 per cent of households), eggs (70 per cent) and milk (52 per cent) (Mason and Jayne, 2009). Big traditional marketplaces (with hundreds or thousands of traders) play a key role in food retail in African cities, and there is a wide range of other types of outlets, such as *spaza* shops, kiosks and *ka* tables, that cater to the different needs of residents (in terms of affordability, variety, quality, quantity, etc.). The urban food environment of African cities is transforming rapidly, however, with the dramatic expansion of supermarkets. This expansion of supermarkets is linked to the nutrition transition towards highly processed foods, which is still underway in Africa. While 'traditional' foods still dominate, there is an increasing growth in the sale and consumption of items like sugar-sweetened beverages, potato chips and sweets (which are, respectively, the third, seventh and ninth most commonly sold food items in Kisumu) (Opiyo, Ogindo and Fuseini, 2018).

Kisumu in Kenya is an example of a secondary city, and represents many of the key characteristics of urban food environments in African cities. It was founded in 1901 by the British as a railway terminus port (Anyumba, 1995), and now is the third-largest city in Kenya, with a population of about 500,000 people (Nodalis Conseil, 2013). Kisumu has a vast range of informal food outlets, ranging from big markets to house shops and pavement traders, and has had a rapid recent increase in supermarkets. Most residents of Kisumu purchase food from informal outlets: a survey of 841 households in Kisumu (across a cross-section of income groups) found that 82 per cent of households purchased food from informal house shops at least five days a week, 75 per cent of households purchased food from other types of informal outlets (kiosks, tuck-shops, traders and hawkers) at least five days a week, 25 per cent of households purchased food from informal markets at least five days per week, and only 7 per cent of households purchased food from supermarkets at least five days a week (although 40 per cent of households purchased food from supermarkets at least once a week) (Opiyo et al., 2018). In addition, 45 per cent of households were severely food-insecure, and a further 21 per cent were moderately food-insecure (Opiyo et al., 2018).

Physically, the urban food environment can be conceptualised as a complex configuration of food outlets (shops, markets, street vendors, etc.) consisting of the following main elements:

- Nodes: Traditional marketplaces (which can have thousands of traders), shopping malls, and clusters of formal or informal shops and traders. Formal and informal trading activities are intertwined, often with a symbiotic relationship (for example, informal sellers of fresh fruit and vegetables are often found outside formal supermarkets).
- Lines of formal and informal food outlets and traders along major transport routes in various formal informal structures (which may be permanent or temporary, and which often only operate at particular times of the day).
- Dispersed pattern of formal and informal food outlets and traders, usually in residential areas. Many outlets take the form of a 'house shop', a dwelling that is also used as a shop.
- Mobile food vendors that move around within and between areas.

These patterns are overlaid on the typical spatial patterns of African cities. Kisumu shows many of the key spatial features of African cities. At the core of the city area is the colonial city, with a grid pattern. The central business district (CBD) is here, with a concentration of commercial activities. An industrial area and some formal residential areas are adjacent to the CBD. Most supermarkets and formal shops are also located here, particularly in the CBD, but also along major transport routes and at major interchanges. The main marketplaces are also located here. In 2009, 16 per cent of the population of Kisumu lived in the colonial core (Nodalis Conseil, 2013). Surrounding the historical core of Kisumu is a zone of informal settlements, which forms a continuous belt (usually referred to as the 'slum belt'). Large numbers of informal shops are located here, and in 2009, 42 per cent of the population of Kisumu lived in these unplanned areas (Nodalis Conseil, 2013). Finally, there is a peri-urban zone, largely characterised by agriculture, but with dispersed development, much of which falls outside formal planning approval processes. In 2009, 42 per cent of the population of the city of Kisumu lived in these peri-urban areas (Nodalis Conseil, 2013).

The survey of food retailers in Kisumu was undertaken in the main street in the CBD, two key markets (Kibuye Market and Jubilee Market) and Nyalenda, one of the largest informal settlements in the city. A total of 2,166 food outlets were surveyed (this information is from the unpublished raw survey data). Although not representative of the city as a whole, the numbers of different types of food retail outlets give a sense of the diversity of the food environment:

- Two big markets with a total of 697 traders with stalls or stands;
- Nine large supermarkets;
- 212 small 'formal' shops (sometimes called 'superettes');
- 340 'informal' shops (kiosks or 'tuck shops');
- 139 house shops;
- 366 street vendors (typically with their goods on a table or on the pavement);
- 210 mobile vendors.

The key elements of the physical urban food environment are discussed below: traditional marketplaces, supermarkets, informal shops, street food vendors and the broader urban food environment in which food outlets are located.

Traditional marketplaces

Traditional marketplaces are a key part of the food environment of African cities, selling essential foodstuffs such as maize, dried fish, fruit and vegetables. The infrastructure of marketplaces can vary enormously. In Kisumu, for example, there are three large metropolitan markets (Jubilee Market, Fish Market, Kibuye Market), sixteen smaller urban markets and ten peri-urban markets (Nodalis Conseil, 2013). These range from the relatively well-equipped Jubilee Market near the centre of the city, through fairly basic markets such as the Manyatta Peace Market, to largely informal markets like Kibuye Market.

Kibuye Market has approximately 7,000 traders (in a mix of shops, kiosks, stalls and open-air traders), while Jubilee Market has about 2,000 traders (Onyango et al., 2013). Market associations generally play an important role in managing marketplaces in Africa (King, 2006; Porter, Lyon and Potts, 2007). They 'control the selling space and can therefore exclude others and have wider effects on the vegetable production and marketing system' (Lyon, 2003: 20). In Maputo, for example, 'the market committees provide infrastructure (water, toilets, etc.), maintenance and security services, and organise cleaning in their respective markets ... The committees also act as the principal regulators in the markets' (Lindell, 2008: 1889). Local governments also usually play a role in managing marketplaces, partially because trader fees can be a significant source of local government revenue (King, 2006). As most local governments lack adequate power to plan, regulate and provide infrastructure and services, this role is often limited to collecting fees (Meagher, 2011).

Jubilee Market in Kisumu is a typical example. Kisumu City collects fees from these traders on a daily or monthly basis: at the Jubilee Market, for example, the fee is 30 Kenyan shillings per day for traders outside the market (collected every day) and 350–600 Kenyan shillings per month for stalls inside the market (paid monthly to the city) – but provides relatively little in return (other than security) (Smit, 2016). In addition to this fee, all delivery vehicles pay an unloading fee for each delivery. Market fees in Kisumu are a significant part of local government revenue, typically making up about 10 per cent of Kisumu City's local revenue (Opiyo, Ogindo and Fuseini, 2018). The Jubilee Market traders' associations collect additional fees to provide services, including sanitation and cleaning.

Supermarkets
Over the past two decades there has been a rapid increase in supermarkets in African cities (Abrahams, 2010; Crush and Frayne, 2011; Reardon et al., 2003; Reardon, Timmer and Berdegué, 2004; Reardon, Henson and Berdegué 2007; Weatherspoon and Reardon, 2003). For example, between 1995 and 2012 Shoprite Checkers, a South African supermarket chain, opened 131 supermarkets in sixteen different African countries outside South Africa (Battersby and Peyton, 2014). In Kisumu, the number of supermarkets has grown rapidly over the past two decades, to about twenty. Formerly, supermarkets were situated only in the CBD, but now there are a growing number located in or near residential areas (Hayombe, Owino and Awuor, 2018).

In some cases, supermarkets play an important role in the food strategies of low-income residents. Fieldwork in Khayelitsha in Cape Town, South Africa, showed that households generally do their major (weekly or monthly) grocery shopping at one of the local shopping malls in

Khayelitsha or neighbouring Mitchells Plain (Smit et al., 2016). Larger shopping rounds usually consist of canned food, flour, rice and sometimes meat. Several respondents in the informal settlement of Taiwan in Khayelitsha said that they did their shopping at the Site B Mall: they travelled there by train, and then they take a minibus taxi back. For residents who shop at the much closer Thembani Shopping Centre, it is a twenty-five-minute walk, but as another respondent added, 'For an elderly person it can even take an hour and a half' (Smit et al., 2016: 200).

In general, the proportion of households that obtain their food from supermarkets is fairly low in most African cities, especially among low-income groups. For example, the Urban Consumption Survey in Zambia found that only 12 per cent of all households bought staple foods (wheat, sorghum, millet and cassava flour, maize meal, rice, samp, pasta, bread, sugar, cassava and potatoes) at supermarkets. The proportion of households shopping at supermarkets varies considerably by income group. For example, in Zambia in 2007–8, 28 per cent of households in the upper income quintile bought staple foods at supermarkets, compared with only 1 per cent of the lowest income quintile (Mason and Jayne, 2009).

Informal shops

Informal shops (known by a variety of names, such as '*spaza* shops' and 'tuck shops') are a very common type of food outlet in African cities. They can either be in purpose-built structures (usually 'informal' in the sense that they do not have planning permission or comply with building regulations) or within dwellings in residential areas. In Kisumu, for example, about 50 per cent of food retail outlets are estimated to be outside of formally zoned retail space (Opiyo, Ogindo and Fuseini, 2018).

Informal shops play an important role in household food strategies in that they sell food in very small quantities and provide credit, so that many households depend on them for their daily purchases, whereas they would often do their major shopping of bulk foodstuffs at supermarkets (Smit et al., 2016). In Kisumu, 52 per cent of informal food traders offer credit (Opiyo, Ogindo and Fuseini, 2018).

Also common in many cities are unregulated alcohol outlets and taverns (called 'shebeens' in South Africa and some other countries). In the Western Cape province in 2010 there were an estimated 20,000 to 35,000 shebeens, compared with 7,538 officially licensed alcohol outlets

(Smit, 2014). These unregulated outlets do not comply with official liquor laws such as trading hours and legal drinking age.

Street food vendors
Street food vendors play an important role in providing affordable cooked food to low-income urban residents (Dixon et al., 2007; Njaya, 2014; Steyn et al., 2014; Van't Riet et al., 2001). However, they generally do not have any suitable infrastructure (shelter from the elements, energy, water, etc.), and are frequently subject to clampdowns and evictions (Devas, 2001; King, 2006; Potts, 2007; Setsabi, 2006). In Kisumu, there have been frequent attempts to relocate street traders from the CBD to designated trading areas (Opiyo, Ogindo and Fuseini, 2018).

The broader urban environment
Over and above the location of different types of food outlet, the broader urban environment can have also a key impact on the food environment, mainly in terms of infrastructure and shelter and the extent of urban agriculture.

Large proportions of residents of African cities live in informal settlements without adequate shelter or basic services, which makes the storage and preparation of food difficult and can cause health risks. In 2014, an estimated 56 per cent of sub-Saharan Africa's urban population lived in informal settlements or other types of slum, in other words areas lacking adequate housing and services. The number of households living in slums in sub-Saharan Africa has been growing steadily, from an estimated 111 million in 1995 to 201 million in 2015 (UN-Habitat, 2016).

Fieldwork in Cape Town showed that residents who lived in informal settlements without access to electricity had to carefully strategise about how to keep perishable food fresh. They either had to buy electricity (illegally) from neighbours or ask neighbours with electricity and refrigerators to store food for them. Often, however, this led to conflict. Other residents who stored food in plastic containers were at risk of the food being eaten by rodents (Smit et al., 2016).

Many African cities have fairly inefficient transport networks and linkages. Most food is transported by road, with trucks used to transport bulky items and large volumes, while smaller quantities of food are transported by buses, *matatus* (minibus taxis) and even *boda bodas* (motorcycle taxis) (Sibanda and Von Blottnitz, 2018). With the exception of major roads between cities, the road system is often not conducive to the transport of foods, complicating supply chains from rural hinterlands to cities. The net result is that imported foods can be cheaper than locally produced foods. For example, in Kisumu, imported frozen Nile perch and tilapia are cheaper than locally caught fish from Lake Victoria (Sibanda and Von Blottnitz, 2018).

The importance of urban agriculture varies considerably between cities and countries in Africa, and is often quite limited (Crush, Hovorka and Tevera, 2011; Zezza and Tasciotti, 2010). It is important to note that there are different types of urban agriculture in Africa, with different dynamics. The distinction between rainy-season urban agriculture and dry-season urban agriculture is particularly important; the example of Lusaka, Zambia, shows that dry-season urban agriculture requires permanent access to land and sources of water and is therefore often dominated by higher-income households, whereas rainy-season agriculture is more likely to be undertaken by low-income households (Drescher, 1999).

While significant numbers of urban households are engaged in urban agriculture, their contribution to food security is usually fairly minor. For example in Zambia in 2015, 17.9 per cent of households in urban areas were engaged in agriculture activities (maize was overwhelmingly the main crop grown), but the monetary value of own food production by urban households as a share of total expenditure was only 3.5 per cent (Central Statistical Office, Republic of Zambia, 2016). Given that, on average, urban households in Zambia spent 37.4 per cent of their monthly outgoings on food, urban-agriculture own production accounted for less than 10 per cent of urban food consumption in terms of the estimated financial value of food consumed (Central Statistical Office, Republic of Zambia, 2016). Similarly in Kisumu, Kenya, only 15 per cent of households who live in the city are involved in urban agriculture (Opiyo et al., 2018).

Food environments and health

Food environment research in the global north has largely been 'in response to the high prevalence of obesity and associated nutrition related non-communicable diseases' (Turner et al., 2017). As a result, the findings generally highlight that 'unhealthy food environments foster unhealthy diets through the widespread availability of cheap, highly palatable, heavily promoted, energy-dense and nutrient-poor foods' (Swinburn et al., 2013: 25). As shown above, however, food environments in African cities are extremely complex, and the key issues are food security and malnutrition (including persistent maternal and child undernutrition) as well as the emerging rapid increases in obesity- and nutrition-related non-communicable diseases (Turner et al., 2017).

The food environment of African cities influences food security, nutrition and health in a variety of ways. For example, the location and type of food outlets influence the availability and accessibility of food in particular areas. Similarly, the extent of urban agriculture may also have an effect on the availability and accessibility of food. The lack of provision of infrastructure for traders and street food vendors may influence food safety. Shelter and infrastructure conditions in residential areas can affect the ability to store food and to prepare and consume food in healthy conditions. In many cases, the resulting food environments are unconducive to food security and healthy diets, contributing to low levels of food security combined with unhealthy diets.

Location and type of food outlets, and access to food

The location and type of food outlets can influence the availability and accessibility of food. In cities of the global north, low-income areas are often characterised by low numbers of food outlets that sell healthy food. These areas have been conceptualised as 'food deserts' (for example, Shaw, 2006). Extending the metaphor, Bridle-Fitzpatrick (2015) has identified 'food swamps' (areas with high levels of unhealthy food) and 'food oases' (areas with high levels of healthy foods). The concepts of food deserts and food swamps are linked to the 'obesogenic environment thesis', that is, that certain environments can promote sedentary behaviour and unhealthy diets, thus resulting in higher levels of obesity (e.g. Hill and Peters, 1998; Lake and Townshend, 2006; Townshend and Lake, 2009). Low-income residential areas in many African cities can be characterised as food swamps rather than food deserts, in that they have a large number of food outlets that, although fresh fruit and vegetables are still widely available, increasingly sell highly processed foods (Frayne and McCordic, 2018). The net result is 'poor, often informal, urban neighbourhoods characterised by high food insecurity and low dietary diversity, with multiple market and non-market food sources but variable household access to food' (Battersby and Crush, 2014: 143).

The impact of the rapid increase in supermarkets in African cities on food security and health is poorly understood, but it is possible that in certain cases it can have a negative impact on dietary patterns and food security. For example, a comparison of Blantyre, Malawi, and Gaberone, Botswana, suggests that the shift from local production of food and a largely informal retail sector to formal supermarkets with international supply chains may result in decreased levels of food security (Riley and Legwegoh, 2014).

Urban agriculture
The relationship of urban agriculture to urban food security and nutritional health is disputed. While some authors (e.g. Lee-Smith, 2010; Maxwell, Levin and Csete, 1998) suggest that urban agriculture has a tangible and beneficial effect on urban food security and health, other authors (e.g. Frayne, McCordic and Shilomboleni, 2014: 187) are of the view that there is 'no significant relationship' between urban agriculture and urban food security and health, as low-income households are usually constrained in access to land and other resources necessary to undertake urban agriculture, and high-income households (who are already food-secure) often tend to participate and benefit more.

Food safety
There are numerous studies that show how inadequate access to water and sanitation and inadequate refuse removal can result in the contamination of food (Barro et al., 2006; Gadaga et al., 2008; Muyanja et al., 2011; Umoh and Odoba, 1999). For example, a study of poultry meat sold at markets in Maputo, Mozambique, found that all the samples purchased were contaminated with faecal matter and had the potential to cause diarrhoea (Cambaza dos Muchangos et al., 2015). A study of street food vendors in Tshwane, South Africa, found that vendors generally followed good hygiene practices, but that the overall environment in which they cooked and sold food resulted in the contamination of food: 'Unavailability of potable water and lack of proper infrastructure for the production of safe food has led to the quality of street-vended ready-to-eat chicken being contaminated by faecal and environmental contaminants and pathogenic organisms' (Oguttu et al., 2015: 202).

In addition to the risks to the safety of the food, many risks are associated with producing and preparing food, for example those from using 'heat generated by unprocessed biofuels and residual oil products'

(Clancy, 2008: 467). The use of waste timber for wood fuel can also expose those who cook food with it to high levels of arsenic (Niyobuhungiro and von Blottnitz, 2013).

Although studies of food safety in Africa have largely focused on food traders, the same sorts of issues would often apply in residential areas without adequate access to water and sanitation and safe forms of energy supply. In the informal settlement of Taiwan in Cape Town, for example, in theory five households have to share a communal toilet, but many of these toilets are kept locked (and thus are inaccessible to other households) and many are in a state of disrepair (e.g. with missing doors) (Smit et al., 2016). This inadequate provision of sanitation is a serious health hazard. Also contributing to the problem is that water has to be collected from communal standpipes and has to be stored in containers, and therefore is at risk of contamination.

Another issue that can influence food safety is solid waste. Solid waste is a by-product of the food system, and uncollected solid waste can have a negative impact on food safety and health, attracting flies and polluting water. In general, fairly low proportions of solid waste are collected in African cities. For example, in Kisumu it is estimated that only between 20 and 35 per cent of solid waste is collected (either directly by the city or by private collectors who sell their services to companies and institutions), leaving about 65-80 per cent (of which most is organic waste) uncollected (Sibanda, Obange and Awuor, 2017).

Creating food environments that are conducive to food security and better health

Currently, food environments in African cities are generally not conducive to food security and healthy diets, but there are possibilities for improving food environments to promote food security and healthy dietary patterns. The key levers for creating food environments that are conducive to food security and better health are land-use zoning; the provision of infrastructure provision; and improving the governance of urban food systems.

Land-use zoning

Land-use zoning has a major impact on food environments, in that it determines where food retail and urban agriculture can legally take place. Although large parts of African cities often, in practice, fall outside such zoning schemes, many key parts of them are subject to the enforcement of land-use zoning. While land-use zoning is a less important tool here than in cities of the global north, it can still have a significant influence on the shaping of urban food environments.

Following conventional urban planning practice, space officially set aside for retail activity is usually in central business districts and community shopping centres and along activity streets. Over the past two decades there has been an increase in shopping malls in African cities, linked to the rapid growth of supermarkets. There is a need to set aside accessible locations for food outlets and to work with shopping mall developers to ensure that informal traders are not excluded from shopping malls. This is hindered by the lack of capacity and resources. For example, Kitwe City Council in Zambia, responsible for a city with a population of about 470,000 people, in 2009 had only nine urban planners and 'just a few old paper maps, which are outdated and inadequate for effective development planning and monitoring in the city' (UN-Habitat, 2009: 9).

Land-use zoning also has an impact on urban agriculture. Part of the reason for many African cities having fairly low levels of urban agriculture is that most African national and local governments are intolerant of urban agriculture, seeing it as incompatible with their 'modernist' visions of what cities should look like (Simatele and Binns, 2008). There needs to be recognition of the need to set aside land for urban agriculture in appropriate areas within cities. In addition, support is needed for low-income households to engage in urban agriculture, for example, with regard to inputs, extension services, credit and financial access, production and marketing infrastructure, and knowledge (Frayne et al., 2014).

Provision of infrastructure

In addition to being a socio-economic right, the provision of infrastructure has a major impact on the food environment. Water, sanitation and energy infrastructure can influence the preparation and consumption of food, in both collective and household spaces, and transport infrastructure can influence the distribution of food. The preparation and consumption of healthy food are extremely difficult in a context in which adequate water and sanitation and a safe energy supply are absent.

The increased provision of household infrastructure is crucial, and given the large proportion of residents living in informal settlements, upgrading these informal settlements is key. City-region transport infrastructure also needs to be improved to help ensure more efficient local supply networks.

Markets are also a particular area of concern. For example, Chisikone Market in Kitwe plays a key role in the local urban food system, but its approximately 10,000 traders have to sell food in very poor conditions, with inadequate access to water and sanitation, and many parts of the market have little storm water drainage. Providing potable water, sanitation and adequate protection from the elements for markets and informal traders is important for helping to ensure food safety. The provision of infrastructure for street traders is also important, to give protection from the elements, water supply and sanitation, and a safe supply of energy (Smit et al., 2011).

Governance

Linked to land-use zoning and the provision of infrastructure, the challenges of urban governance in many African cities needs to be acknowledged. These include incomplete decentralisation (and in some cases recentralisation), resulting in weak and under-resourced local governments, and the diffusion of power among a range of governance actors, including community groups that play the role of local government in many informal settlements and traditional leaders that often play the role of local government in peri-urban areas (Meagher, 2011; Smit and Pieterse, 2014; UN-Habitat, 2008). There also are high levels of political contestation, often linked to ethnic identity and client–patron relations (Resnick, 2011).

There is an urgent need to bring urban governance actors together in order to develop and implement coherent strategies to improve urban food security (Smit, 2018). Local governance actors need to think explicitly about the governance of urban food systems, through collaborative mechanisms such as multi-stakeholder food policy councils (Haysom, 2015; Pereira and Drimie, 2016; Rocha and Lessa, 2009; Smit, 2016). For example, the Kisumu Action Team brought together different interests in Kisumu (including big business and informal traders) to develop a strategic plan for the city that included the upgrading of marketplaces (Onyango and Obera, 2015).

Civil society organisations have a particularly important role to play in these processes as they generally represent the interests of marginalised groups, who are often excluded from decision-making processes.

A range of civil society organisations are involved in urban food issues, such as non-governmental organisations that are involved in food production and food philanthropy, community-based organisations that operate food programmes for vulnerable populations, and social movements that 'operate on broader political, economic or social issues ranging from land reform to food prices' (Warshawsky, 2016: 310). These civil society organisations need to be brought into formal food governance processes.

Conclusion

The first key point highlighted by this chapter is that the urban food environments of African cities are complex, with large numbers of outlets and traders and a wide range of different types of outlet, and multiple layers of formality and informality.

The second key point is that urban food environments are inadequate in many ways: for example, many informal traders lack basic services, supermarkets are often located in inappropriate areas, and the lack of basic services in low-income residential areas greatly constrains the ability of residents to safely prepare and consume food.

Third, there is a need for proactive inter-sectoral planning to improve urban food environments and ensure that they are more conducive for good health and wellbeing, for example through ensuring that markets and street traders are provided with appropriate infrastructure, that residential areas have adequate basic services (such as water and sanitation) and that suitable land is set aside for urban agriculture where appropriate. In addition, it is essential to develop governance mechanisms and processes that can include a more diverse range of stakeholders, such as informal traders and informal settlement communities, in decision-making processes about urban food environments. The views of informal traders and informal settlement communities are essential in creating better-functioning food environments, but perspectives such as these are often ignored in decision-making.

Fourth, in order to provide an evidence base for planning for urban food environments, there is a need for interdisciplinary and transdisciplinary research on food environments, as this is a complex and multi-faceted issue that cuts across disciplines and sectors. There is a need to explore the interaction of people's foodways and the multiple urban environments they move through, and this should be placed within the broader physical, social, economic and political context of the cities (and rural hinterlands) they live in. We need to move beyond simplistic metaphors such as 'food deserts' (and food swamps and food oases) and understand the complex ways in which urban food environments can affect health-related behaviours and outcomes.

Acknowledgements

This chapter draws on work undertaken as part of the project Consuming Urban Poverty, funded by the Economic and Social Research Council (ESRC), as well as other work undertaken in Cape Town, to highlight the complexity of food environments of African cities and explore possibilities for how food environments that are more conducive to health and wellbeing can be created and sustained.

References

Abrahams, C. (2010). Transforming the region: Supermarkets and the local food economy. *African Affairs*, 109(434): 115–34.

Alkon, A.H., Block, D., Moore, K., Gillis, C., DiNuccio, N., and Chavez, N. (2013). Foodways of the urban poor. *Geoforum*, 48: 126–35.

Anyumba, G. (1995). *Kisumu Town: History of the built form, planning and environment, 1890–1990*. Delft: Delft University Press.

Barro, N., Bello, A.R., Savadogo, A., Ouattara, C.A., Iiboudo, A.J., and. Traoré, A.S. (2006). Hygienic status assessment of dish washing waters, utensils, hands and pieces of money from street food processing sites in Ouagadougou (Burkina Faso). *African Journal of Biotechnology*, 5(11): 1107–12.

Battersby, J., and Crush, J. (2014). Africa's urban food deserts. *Urban Forum*, 25(2): 143–51.

Battersby, J., and Peyton, S. (2014). The geography of supermarkets in Cape Town: Supermarket expansion and food access. *Urban Forum*, 25(2): 153–64.

Battersby, J., and Watson, V. (2018). Addressing food security in African cities. *Nature Sustainability*, 1(4): 153–5.

Bridle-Fitzpatrick, S. (2015). Food deserts or food swamps? A mixed-methods study of local food environments in a Mexican city. *Social Science & Medicine*, 142: 202–13.

Cambaza dos Muchangos, A.B., Roesel, K., McCrindle, C., Matusse, H., Hendrickx, S., Makita, K. and Grace, D. (2015). Informal markets in Mozambique risky for local chicken. In K. Roesel and D. Grace (eds), *Food safety and informal markets: Animal products in sub-Saharan Africa*, 197–200. Abingdon: Routledge.

Cannuscio, C.C., Weiss, E.E., and Asch, D.A. (2010). The contribution of urban foodways to health disparities. *Journal of Urban Health*, 87(3): 381–93.

Caspi, C.E., Sorensen, G. Subramanian, S.V. and Kawachi, I. (2012). The local food environment and diet: A systematic review. *Health & Place*, 18(5): 1172–87.

Central Statistical Office, Republic of Zambia. (2016). *2015 living conditions monitoring survey: Key findings*. Lusaka: Central Statistical Office, Republic of Zambia.

Clancy, J.S. (2008). Urban ecological footprints in Africa. *African Journal of Ecology*, 46 (4): 463–70.

Cobb, L.K., Appel, L.J., Franco, M., Jones-Smith, J.C., Nur, A. and Anderson, C.A.M. (2015). The relationship of the local food environment with obesity: A systematic review of methods, study quality, and results. *Obesity*, 23(7): 1331–44.

Crush, J., and Frayne, B. (2011). Supermarket expansion and the informal food economy in southern African cities: Implications for urban food security. *Journal of Southern African Studies*, 37(4): 781–807.

Crush, J., Hovorka, A., and Tevera, D. (2011). Food security in southern African cities: The place of urban agriculture. *Progress in Development Studies* 11(4): 285–305.

Devas, N. (2001). Does city governance matter for the urban poor? *International Planning Studies*, 6(4): 393–408.

de Zeeuw, H., and Prain, G. (2011). Effects of the global financial crisis and food price hikes of 2007/2008 on the food security of poor urban households. *Urban Agriculture Magazine*, 25: 36–38.

Dixon, J., Omwega, A.M., Friel, S., Burns, C., Donati, K., and Carlisle, R. (2007). The health equity dimensions of urban food systems. *Journal of Urban Health*, 84(1): 118–29.

Doak, C. M., Adair, L.S., Bentley, M., Monteiro, C., and Popkin, B.M. (2004). The dual burden household and the nutrition transition paradox. *International Journal of Obesity*, 29(1): 129–36.

Drescher, A.W. (1999). Urban agriculture in the seasonal tropics: The case of Lusaka, Zambia. In M. Koc, R. MacRae, L.J.A. Mougeot and J. Welsh (eds), *For hunger-proof cities: Sustainable urban food systems*, 67–76. Ottawa: International Development Research Centre.

FAO (2009). *Declaration of the World Summit on Food Security*. Rome: FAO.

FAO (2016). *Influencing food environments for healthy diets*. Rome: FAO.

Frayne, B. and McCordic, C. (2018). Food swamps and poor dietary diversity: Longwave development implications in Southern African cities. *Sustainability*, 10(12), art. 4425.

Frayne, B., McCordic, C., and Shilomboleni, H. (2014). Growing out of poverty: Does urban agriculture contribute to household food security in southern African cities? *Urban Forum*, 25(2): 177–89.

Frayne, B., Pendleton, W., Crush, J., Acquah, B., Battersby-Lennard, J., Bras, E., Chiweza, A., Dlamini, T., Fincham, R., Kroll, F., Leduka, C., Mosha, A., Mulenga, C., Mvula, P., Pomuti, A., Raimundo, I., Rudolph, M., Ruysenaa, S., Simelane, N., Tevera, D., Tsoka, M., Tawodzera, G., and Zanamwe, L. (2010). *The state of urban food insecurity in southern Africa*. Urban Food Security Series 2. Kingston and Cape Town: Queen's University and the African Food Security Urban Network (AFSUN).

Gadaga, T.H., Samende, B.K., Musuna, C., and Chibanda, D. (2008). The microbiological quality of informally vended foods in Harare, Zimbabwe. *Food Control*, 19(8): 829–32.

Glanz, K., Sallis, J.F., Saelens, B.E., and Frank, L.D. (2007). Nutrition environment measures survey in stores (NEMS-S): Development and evaluation. *American Journal of Preventive Medicine*, 32(4): 282–9.

Hansen, K.T., and Vaa, M. (2004). Introduction. In K.T. Hansen and M. Vaa (eds), *Reconsidering informality: Perspectives from urban Africa*, 7–24. Uppsala: Nordiska Afrikainstitutet.

Hayombe, P.O., Owino, F.O., and Awuor, F.O. (2018). Planning and governance of food systems in Kisumu City. In J. Battersby and V. Watson (eds), *Urban food systems, governance and poverty in African cities*, 116–27. London: Routledge.

Haysom, G. (2015). Food and the city: Urban scale food system governance. *Urban Forum*, 26(3): 263–81.

Herforth, A., and Ahmed, S. (2015). The food environment, its effects on dietary consumption, and potential for measurement within agriculture-nutrition interventions. *Food Security*, 7(3): 505–20.

Hill, J.O., and Peters, J.C. (1998). Environmental contributions to the obesity epidemic. *Science*, 280(5368): 1371–74.

Kimani-Murage, E. W., Schofield, L., Wekesah, F., Mohamed, S., Mberu, B., Ettarh, R., Egondi, T., Kyobutungi, C., and Ezeh, A. (2014). Vulnerability to food insecurity in urban slums: Experiences from Nairobi, Kenya. *Journal of Urban Health*, 91(6): 1098–113.

King, R. (2006). Fulcrum of the urban economy: Governance and street livelihoods in Kumasi, Ghana. In A. Brown (ed.), *Contested space: Street trading, public space, and livelihoods in developing cities*, 99–118. Rugby: ITDG Publishing.

Lake, A., and Townshend, T. (2006). Obesogenic environments: Exploring the built and food environments. *Journal of the Royal Society for the Promotion of Health*, 126(6): 262–7.

Lake, A.A., Burgoine, T., Greenhalgh, F., Stamp, E., and Tyrrell, R. (2010). The foodscape: Classification and field validation of secondary data sources. *Health & Place*, 16(4): 666–73.

Lee-Smith, D. (2010). Cities feeding people: An update on urban agriculture in Equatorial Africa. *Environment and Urbanization*, 22(2): 483–99.

Lindell, I. (2008). The multiple sites of urban governance: Insights from an African city. *Urban Studies*, 45(9): 1879–901.

Lyon, F. (2003). Trader associations and urban food systems in Ghana: Institutionalist approaches to understanding urban collective action. *International Journal of Urban and Regional Research*, 27(1), 11–23. doi: 10.1111/1468-2427.00428.

Mason, N.M. and Jayne, T.S. (2009). *Staple food consumption patterns in urban Zambia: Results from the 2007/2008 urban consumption survey*. Food Security Collaborative Policy Briefs 56810. East Lansing: Department of Agricultural, Food, and Resource Economics, Michigan State University.

Maxwell, D., Levin, C., and Csete, J. (1998). Does urban agriculture help prevent malnutrition? Evidence from Kampala. *Food Policy*, 23(5): 411–24.

McKinnon, R.A., Reedy, J., Morrissette, M.A., Lytle, L.A., and Yaroch, A.L. (2009). Measures of the food environment: A compilation of the literature, 1990–2007. *American Journal of Preventive Medicine*, 36(4, Supplement): S124–S133.

Meagher, K. (2011). Informal economies and urban governance in Nigeria: Popular empowerment or political exclusion? *African Studies Review*, 54(02): 47–72.

Muyanja, C., Nayiga, L., Brenda, N., and Nasinyama, G. (2011). Practices, knowledge and risk factors of street food vendors in Uganda. *Food Control*, 22(10): 1551–8.

Niyobuhungiro, R.V., and von Blottnitz, H. (2013). Investigation of arsenic airborne in particulate matter around caterers' wood fires in the Cape Town region. *Aerosol and Air Quality Research*, 13(1): 219–24.

Njaya, T. (2014). Operations of street food vendors and their impact on sustainable urban life in high density suburbs of Harare, in Zimbabwe. *Asian Journal of Economic Modelling*, 2(1): 18–31.

Nodalis Conseil (2013). *Kisumu ISUD Plan – Part 1*. Paris: Nodalis.

Oguttu, J., Roesel, K., McCrindle, C., Hendrickx, S., Makita, K., and Grace, D. (2015). Arrive alive in South Africa: Chicken meat the least to worry about. In K. Roesel and D. Grace (eds), *Food safety and informal markets: Animal products in sub-Saharan Africa*, 202–20. Abingdon: Routledge.

Onyango, G.M., and Obera. B.O. (2015). Tracing Kisumu's path in the co-production of knowledge for urban development. In M. Polk (ed.), *Co-producing knowledge for sustainable cities: Joining forces for change*, 73–97. Abingdon: Routledge.

Onyango, G.M., Wagah, G.G., Omondi, L.A., and Obera, B.O. (2013). *Market places: Experiences from Kisumu City*. Kisumu: Maseno University Press.

Opiyo, P., Ogindo, H., and Fuseini, I. (2018). *Characteristics of the urban food system in Kisumu (Kenya)*. Consuming Urban Poverty Working Paper No. 5. Cape Town: African Centre for Cities.

Opiyo, P., Obange, N., Ogindo, H., and Wagah, G. (2018). *The characteristics, extent and drivers of urban food poverty in Kisumu, Kenya*. Consuming Urban Poverty Working Paper No. 5. Cape Town: African Centre for Cities.

Pereira, L. and Drimie, S. (2016). Governance arrangements for the future food system: Addressing complexity in South Africa. *Environment: Science and Policy for Sustainable Development*, 58(4): 18–31.

Porter, G., Lyon, F., and Potts, D. (2007). Market institutions and urban food supply in West and southern Africa: A review. *Progress in Development Studies*, 7(2): 115–34.

Potts, D. (2007). City life in Zimbabwe at a time of fear and loathing: Urban planning, urban poverty and Operation Murambatsvina. In G. Myers and M. Murray (eds), *Cities in contemporary Africa*, 265–88. New York: Palgrave Macmillan.

Reardon, T., Henson, S., and Berdegué, J. (2007). 'Proactive fast-tracking' diffusion of supermarkets in developing countries: Implications for market institutions and trade. *Journal of Economic Geography*, 7(4): 399–431.

Reardon, T., Timmer, C.P., Barrett, C.B., and Berdegué, J. (2003). The rise of supermarkets in Africa, Asia, and Latin America. *American Journal of Agricultural Economics*, 85(5): 1140–6.

Reardon, T., Timmer, P., and Berdegue, J. (2004). The rapid rise of supermarkets in developing countries: Induced organizational, institutional, and technological change in agrifood systems. *Electronic Journal of Agricultural and Development Economics*, 1(2): 168–83.

Resnick, D. (2011). In the shadow of the city: Africa's urban poor in opposition strongholds. *The Journal of Modern African Studies*, 49(1): 141–66.

Riley, L., and Legwegoh A. (2014). Comparative urban food geographies in Blantyre and Gaborone. *African Geographical Review*, 33(1): 52–66.

Rocha, C., and Lessa, I. (2009). Urban governance for food security: The alternative food system in Belo Horizonte, Brazil. *International Planning Studies*, 14(4): 389–400.

Setsabi, S. (2006). Contest and conflict: Governance and street livelihoods in Maseru, Lesotho. In A. Brown (ed.), *Contested space: Street trading, public space, and livelihoods in developing cities*, 131–52. Rugby: ITDG Publishing.

Shaw, H.J. (2006). Food deserts: Towards the development of a classification. *Geografiska Annaler: Series B, Human Geography*, 88(2): 231–47.

Sibanda, L.K., Obange, N., and Awuor, F.O. (2017). Challenges of solid waste management in Kisumu, Kenya. *Urban Forum*, 28(4): 387–402.

Sibanda, L.K., and von Blottnitz, H. (2018). *Food systems description – Kisumu*. Consuming Urban Poverty Field Report No.1. Cape Town: African Centre for Cities.

Simatele, D.M., and Binns, T. (2008). Motivation and marginalization in African urban agriculture: The case of Lusaka, Zambia. *Urban Forum*, 19(1): 1–21.

Smit, W. (2014). Discourses of alcohol: Reflections on key issues influencing the regulation of Shebeens in Cape Town. *South African Geographical Journal*, 96 (1): 60–80.

Smit, W. (2016). Urban governance and urban food systems in Africa: Examining the linkages. *Cities*, 58: 80–6.

Smit, W. (2018). Current urban food governance and planning in Africa. In J. Battersby and V. Watson (eds), *Urban food systems governance and poverty in African cities*, 94–103. Abingdon: Routledge.

Smit, W., de Lannoy, A., Dover, R.V.H., Lambert, E.V., Levitt, N., and Watson, V. (2016). Making unhealthy places: The built environment and non-communicable diseases in Khayelitsha, Cape Town. *Health & Place*, 39: 196–203.

Smit, W., Hancock, T., Kumaresen, J., Santos-Burgoa, C., Sánchez-Kobashi Meneses, R., and Friel, S. (2011). Toward a research and action agenda on urban planning/design and health equity in cities in low and middle-income countries. *Journal of Urban Health*, 88(5): 875–85.

Smit, W., and Pieterse, E. (2014). Decentralisation and institutional reconfiguration in urban Africa. In S. Parnell and E. Pieterse (eds), *Africa's urban revolution: Policy pressures*, 148–66. London: Zed Books.

Spence, J.C., Cutumisu, N., Edwards, J., Raine, K.D., and Smoyer-Tomic, K. (2009). Relation between local food environments and obesity among adults. *BMC Public Health*, 9, art. 192.

Steyn, N.P., Mchiza, Z., Hill, J., Davids, Y.D., Venter, I., Hinrichsen, E., Opperman, M., Rumbelow, J., and Jacobs, P. (2014). Nutritional contribution of street foods to the diet of people in developing countries: A systematic review. *Public Health Nutrition*, 17(6): 1363–74.

Swinburn, B., Vandevijvere, S., Kraak, V., Sacks, G., Snowdon, W., Hawkes, C., Barquera, S., Friel, S., Kelly, B., Kumanyika, S., L'Abbé, M., Lee, A., Lobstein, T., Ma, J., Macmullan, J., Mohan, S., Monteiro, C., Neal, B., Rayner, M., Sanders, D., and Walker, C. (2013). Monitoring and benchmarking government policies and actions to improve the healthiness of food environments: A proposed government healthy food environment policy index. *Obesity Reviews*, 14(S1): 24–37.

Townshend, T., and Lake, A.A. (2009). Obesogenic urban form: Theory, policy and practice. *Health & Place*, 15(4): 909–16.

Townshend, T., and Lake, A. (2017). Obesogenic environments: Current evidence of the built and food environments. *Perspectives in Public Health*, 137(1): 38–44.

Turner, C., Kadiyala, S., Aggarwal, A., Coates, J., Drewnowski, A., Hawkes, C., Herforth, A., Kalamatianou, S., and Walls, H. (2017). *Concepts and methods for food environment research in low and middle income countries.*

Agriculture, Nutrition and Health Academy Food Environments Working Group (ANH-FEWG) Technical Brief. London: Innovative Methods and Metrics for Agriculture and Nutrition Actions (IMMANA).

Umoh, V. J., and Odoba, M.B. (1999). Safety and quality evaluation of street foods sold in Zaria, Nigeria. *Food Control*, 10(1): 9–14.

UN-Habitat (2008). *The state of African cities 2008: A framework for addressing urban challenges in Africa*. Nairobi: UN-Habitat.

UN-Habitat (2009). *Zambia: Kitwe urban profile*. Nairobi: UN-Habitat.

UN-Habitat (2016). *Urbanization and development: Emerging futures – World cities report 2016*. Nairobi: UN-Habitat.

Van't Riet, H., den Hartog, A., Mwangi, A., Mwadime, R., Foeken, D., and van Staveren, W. (2001). The role of street foods in the dietary pattern of two low-income groups in Nairobi. *European Journal of Clinical Nutrition*, 55(7): 562–70.

Warshawsky, D.N. (2016). Civil society and the governance of urban food systems in sub-Saharan Africa. *Geography Compass*, 10(7): 305–18.

Weatherspoon, D.D., and Reardon, T. (2003). The rise of supermarkets in Africa: Implications for agrifood systems and the rural poor. *Development Policy Review*, 21(3): 333–55.

Zenk, S. N., Schulz, A.J., BIsrael, B.A., James, S.A., Bao, S., and Wilson, M.L. (2005). Neighborhood racial composition, neighborhood poverty, and the spatial accessibility of supermarkets in metropolitan Detroit. *American Journal of Public Health*, 95(4): 660–7.

Zezza, A., and Tasciotti, L. (2010). Urban agriculture, poverty, and food security: Empirical evidence from a sample of developing countries. *Food Policy*, 35(4): 265–73.

7

Urban mental health and the moral economies of suffering in a 'broken city': reinventing depression among Rio de Janeiro urban dwellers

Leandro David Wenceslau and Francisco Ortega

Urban living is frequently regarded as a source of both benefits (e.g. access to public services and labour market) and risks (e.g. violence and pollution) to its inhabitants. The so-called urban paradox (Iossifova, Doll and Gasparatos, 2018) has engaged researchers from different disciplines interested in how urban dwellers cope with life in cities and whether, and in what conditions, the benefits outweigh the risks. In urban health research it is no different. While city living is associated with health hazards resulting from risk factors in the urban social or physical environments (Grant, 2018; Grant et al., 2009; Kjellstrom et al., 2007), it is also associated with better access to health care, education and employment (Gruebner et al., 2017).

Several studies show a negative correlation between mental health and urban living. Mood and anxiety disorders are more prevalent among city dwellers (who have a 40 per cent increased risk of depression and more than 20 per cent for anxiety) than among residents of rural areas, and there is a higher risk of schizophrenia for people who grew up in cities in comparison to rural areas (Peen et al., 2010; Krabbendam and van Os, 2005; van Os, Pedersen and Mortensen, 2004). In Brazil, a nationwide study of depression shows a 50 per cent higher prevalence among individuals living in urban areas (Munhoz et al., 2016).

While city–rural comparison constitutes one area of study in urban health research (the other two being comparisons between cities and within cities: see Galea and Vlahov, 2005), in this chapter we are more interested in differences within cities, and more specifically we explore the care offered to people with depressive symptoms in primary health care facilities in the city of Rio de Janeiro.

Among the risk factors for mental health originating from the urban social environment, the concentration of low socio-economic status is the most important and shows the most consistent association. Poverty and deprivation are associated with greater risk of depression and schizophrenia (Galea et al., 2007; Rapp et al., 2015). Moreover, urban inequity is related to levels of insecurity and violence in cities, factors that directly influence mental wellbeing (Stephens, Carrizo and Ostadtaghizaddeh, 2016).

Brazilian cities exhibit high levels of urban inequity, and results from the São Paulo Megacity Mental Health Survey statistically associate those living in areas with medium and high levels of income inequality with increased risk of depression relative to those living in areas with low levels of income inequality (Chiavegatto Filho et al., 2013). Moreover, according to the Brazilian National Health Survey, in 2013, the proportion of Brazilians who did not receive any treatment for depression was 78.8 per cent, while 14.1 per cent received only pharmacological treatments. Access to care is scarce and above all unequal, with poor people and those living in low-resource areas having less access to mental health care than other people (Lopes et al., 2016). Beyond the problem of access, there are several reasons for the limited engagement with mental health care among low-income populations. These include the failure to acknowledge that one has a significant problem, the belief that the disorder will resolve itself spontaneously, a desire to deal with the problem by oneself or not knowing where to search for help, a perception that the treatments available are not efficient or are deleterious, and stigma-related barriers (Silva et al., 2013: 288; Van Beljouw et al., 2010; Thornicroft, 2007; Corrigan, 2004).

Understanding these disparities is an important aspect of developing effective mental health interventions, but so is rejecting 'one-size-fits-all' approaches. Global Mental Health initiatives recognise alternative, community-based and culturally sensitive approaches from low- to middle-income countries, and reject standardised approaches to treating depression and other conditions (Patel and Saxena, 2014). And yet there is an important tension between the need for locally appropriate and participatory approaches on the one hand, and on the other the dismissal of those approaches and interventions when they fail to match the standards of evidence-based practices and interventions, particularly efforts to 'scale up' and generalise those interventions (Ortega, 2018).

Conditions like depression, with which we deal specifically in this chapter, have socio-economic and environmental determinants for wealthy city dwellers which differ from those for people living in low-income neighbourhoods or urban refugees. Depression can have different manifestations for these individuals, and therefore approaches by mental health professionals have to be differentiated (Stephens, Carrizo and Ostadtaghizaddeh, 2016). These differences call for socially attuned interventions and policies that address the specific cultural and mental health needs of urban dwellers (Caracci, 2006).

Brazil can be considered the country with the highest prevalence of common mental disorders in the world, with the second-highest prevalence of depressive disorders in Latin America (5.8 per cent) and the highest prevalence in the world of anxiety disorders (9.3 per cent) (World Health Organization (WHO), 2017). The São Paulo Megacity Mental Health Survey has shown that this scenario is even more serious in the larger Brazilian urban centres, with a prevalence of 19.9 per cent for anxiety disorders and 11 per cent for mood disorders (9.4 per cent for major depressive disorders) in the Metropolitan Region of São Paulo (Andrade et al., 2012).[1] In addition to the global controversies surrounding the diagnostic criteria of mental disorders and the epidemiological instruments used to measure them, these data point to the significant levels of moral, emotional and social suffering among residents of the Brazilian metropolises. This suffering is associated both with difficulties in their social life and with a lack of capacity to manage other health conditions, especially chronic conditions such as diabetes, obesity, hypertension and chronic respiratory diseases. This chapter focuses on the sociocultural processes and social determinants involved in engendering this urban landscape of suffering, and the local responses to these difficulties within public health services.

'Hill' and 'asphalt' in Rio de Janeiro

Rio de Janeiro is the second largest city in Brazil, with more than 6 million inhabitants. The city has experienced varying fortunes in recent years, from hosting international mega-events such as the 2014 FIFA World Cup and the 2016 Olympics to being one of the main victims of the political disputes that since 2014 have created a serious economic crisis in Brazil. Paradoxes and social divisions permeate the social organisation of the Rio de Janeiro population, which has been studied in the last few decades mainly through the lens of the divide between 'hill' and 'asphalt'.[2] Comparing the reactions of different social strata of the city to an *arrastão* – a series of simultaneous assaults carried out on a beach in Rio de Janeiro – the Brazilian journalist Zuenir Ventura described Rio de Janeiro in 1994 as a 'broken city' (Ventura, 1994). The spatial and housing division is associated with differences in income and access to social rights. In Rio de Janeiro, this division takes on a particular character, because of its peculiar territorial overlap – given the geographical proximity between the 'hills' and the more urbanised areas of 'asphalt' below – and the intense social conflicts resulting from the structural violence produced by social inequality and armed violence catalysed by illegal drug trafficking.

While other cities, such as São Paulo, could be viewed as 'surrounded cities' because of the peripheralisation of poverty, in Rio de Janeiro luxury buildings are situated within a few blocks, or even metres, of hills lacking even basic sanitation, with low income and educational levels. Between 1996 and 2008 the Gini coefficient for social inequality remained stable in Rio de Janeiro and poverty levels actually increased, in contrast to the picture at the national level, where both poverty and inequality rates reduced during this period (Neri, 2010).

This chapter analyses recent transformations in public mental health care in Rio de Janeiro from an ethnographic perspective. At the heart of these transformations was the significant expansion of the Family Health Strategy (FHS) – the primary health care model within the Brazilian universal public health system (SUS in Portuguese) – within the city (Paim et al., 2011; Macinko and Harris, 2015). In 2009 less than 7 per cent of the population in Rio de Janeiro City was assisted by a family health team. In December 2017 the proportion had risen to around 70.6 per cent. In absolute numbers, this means that, over eight years, approximately 4 million additional residents were absorbed into the FHS system (Ministério da Saúde, 2016; Prado Junior, 2015; Harzeim, 2013). This care includes mental health approaches and initial therapeutics offered by a general practitioner, especially for the most prevalent disorders: depression, anxiety and/or use and abuse of alcohol, tobacco and other drugs. Alongside the expansion of primary care coverage, the municipal health secretary instituted Family Medicine as the largest Brazilian programme of medical residency (currently with 150 positions), in addition to supporting the expansion of programmes in other institutions. In 2010 Rio de Janeiro had sixteen yearly residency positions for Family Medicine. By 2016 that number had increased to 202 (Soranz, 2014).

One of the authors of this chapter (Wenceslau) worked as a family physician in Rio de Janeiro City in 2013 and identified, through informal conversations and in his daily work routine, the presence of discourses and practices among FHS professionals that sought to integrate social and cultural influences into their diagnosis and proposed treatment of individuals dealing with mental illness. To the health care professionals, there were differences both in how mental issues were presented (that is, the narratives and behaviour of patients and family members) and in their causes between those living in the 'hill' and those in the 'asphalt'. Thus we developed an exploratory ethnographic study in order to evaluate how this division was used to both understand and address mental suffering among the Rio de Janeiro population.

In order to carry out the study, we selected a family health unit in the north zone of Rio de Janeiro responsible for the care of approximately 25,000 people, comprising eight teams and covering areas both in the 'hill' and in the 'asphalt'. The unit was located in a middle-class neighbourhood, whose social development index ranked between the tenth and twentieth highest of the 158 neighbourhoods in Rio de Janeiro (Cavallieri and Peres Lopes, 2008). We interviewed thirteen Family Medicine physicians and, of these, selected six to be followed for three months, through participant observation of their activities during consultations, home visits and work meetings. During this period, we also interviewed and closely followed the assessment and treatment of twenty-two patients, twelve of whom lived in the 'hill' and ten in the 'asphalt'.

We also chose to work with a 'mental health problem' lens, a native category, used by Family Medicine physicians in order to group together the most common accounts and manifestations of suffering that they designated as 'mental'. In view of the setting, a public primary health care facility, we focused our investigation on how 'depressive symptoms' were addressed. Among the most common mental disorders, depression and anxiety are considered the most prevalent in the general population and in primary care (Lim et al., 2018; Steel et al., 2014), with depression being the single largest contributor to non-fatal health loss (WHO, 2017). Studies and documents that guide the integration of mental health into primary health care establish that its professionals may and must be capable of identifying and offering resolutive care to patients with mild and moderate depression and also of recognising and following, with specialised mental health care, more severe cases (WHO and World Organization of Family Doctors (WONCA), 2008; WONCA, 2018; WHO, 2016; Wahlbeck, 2015).

In the FHS, professionals are distributed in teams that are each responsible, on average, for 3,500 to 4,000 people (Ministério da Saúde, 2012; Ministério da Saúde, 2017). The six physicians we followed were members of four different teams. We were able to identify an initial repercussion of the division between 'hill' and 'asphalt', as defined by these teams. Among the four teams we followed, one was dedicated exclusively to the poorer community in the region, while the other three were responsible for the middle-class population. The professionals themselves referred to the poorer community as the 'hill' and to the middle-class population as the 'asphalt'.

To these professionals, there were important differences between the depressive symptoms of these two populations. In the interviews, they stated that the 'hill' population was unlikely to present isolated cases of depression, rather presenting mixed experiences of depressive and anxious symptoms and important bodily manifestations (such as diffuse pains, dizziness and fatigue). Patients from the 'asphalt', on the other hand, in the view of the physicians, presented more typical cases of depression, characterised by symptoms of profound sadness and withdrawal from social interaction.

Health care professionals also acknowledged the importance of social determinants in the production of depressive symptoms and in their evolution. According to them, in the 'hill' people lived more 'within networks', and, as a result, the sorrows and suffering they experienced received greater care from the community, leading those individuals to present manifestations and accounts viewed as 'depressive' less frequently. These 'networks', which worked as mechanisms for social protection and care, were made up of the close supportive relations between neighbours and by the social interaction within different community institutions, such as Evangelical churches, centres of Afro-Brazilian culture and religion, and artistic-cultural associations, such as the community's samba school. On the other hand, the 'asphalt' population had little in the way of networks, with few relationships between neighbours, distance from family members and low participation in other spaces of social interaction.

In the professionals' perception, the depressive symptoms experienced by 'asphalt' inhabitants manifested the social isolation and financial decline that frequently affected them and that recurred among the older segment of this population. The fact that, over the course of their lives, this population was less exposed to social stressors, such as poverty and violence, had, according to the health professionals, rendered the inhabitants 'less resilient' and more susceptible to the development of depressive symptoms when faced with difficulties that, on the other hand, were part of the 'hill' population's everyday lives (for example, unexpected deaths of relatives or friends, lack of food, inadequate housing). However, despite being 'more resilient', when presenting depressive symptoms the 'hill' population did so more intensely, with many bodily manifestations, including frequent incidences of 'syncope' (fainting), as a result of the disruption of nearly all of their social bonds.

To the physicians, 'somatisation' in cases of depression was more common among 'hill' inhabitants than among 'asphalt' inhabitants. This perception is connected with an intense and protracted debate within anthropological studies which, directly or indirectly, has analysed the expansion of public mental health care, including the field's most recent iteration, Global Mental Health (Patel and Prince, 2010). Since the publication of a number of important transcultural psychiatry works such as 'Depression, somatization and the "new cross-cultural psychiatry"' (Kleinman, 1977) and a number of seminal ethnographic studies in various countries – including work on 'nerves' and 'nervousness' in Brazil (Duarte, 1986; Duarte, 1997) – there has been a discussion surrounding the hypothesis that depressive symptoms, especially among lower-income groups or less industrialised populations, could present themselves predominantly as physical or bodily grievances, as local idioms of distress or even as certain culture-bound syndromes (Kleinman and Good, 1985; Jenkins, Kleinman and Good, 1991). This hypothesis was strongly disputed by authors such as Abas et al. (1994) and Patel (2001; Patel et al., 2001), who pointed both to the importance of the presentation of depression through physical symptoms among more elite and industrialised populations and to the identification of psychological manifestations through 'culturally adapted' questionnaires in less Westernised groups. However, controversies remain with regard to the existence of a set of symptoms, however varied in their composition, that can be seen to globally represent a case of depression: critics point to the risk of incurring a categorical fallacy, that is, a selective recognition of manifestations and phenomena produced by the interest in identifying a certain category within a certain social and cultural universe (Haroz et al., 2017; Kirmayer, Gomez-Carrillo and Veissière, 2017). The different perceptions of depressive symptoms among doctors and patients from the 'hill' and those from the 'asphalt' observed in this research are an example of the difficulties in establishing such a pattern.

Therapeutic approaches: 'social networks' and 'patient-centred' consultations

The perceived differences between manifestations of depressive suffering among people from the 'asphalt' and among people from the 'hill' were also translated into distinct emphases in proposed treatments and care, especially through non-pharmacological interventions. The acknowledgement of a 'lack of networks' as one of the main causes of depression in the 'asphalt' led professionals to insist strongly on offering 'unit groups' to those patients. 'Unit groups' were social activities led by health professionals for the purpose of offering spaces for social interaction and learning, such as the 'dance group', 'crafts group', 'wellbeing group' and other, more psychotherapeutic groups, such as the 'cuca fresca' (cool head) group and the 'mental health group', conducted by psychologists. Members of the 'asphalt' population were also more frequently referred for individual psychological assessment and more likely to 'join the queue' for medium- and long-term psychotherapeutic care.

Evaluation by a psychiatrist from the 'matrix support team' was also commonly suggested to the 'asphalt' dwellers by physicians.[3] Many of these patients had at one point had better financial circumstances and had not previously used the public health system, but rather private insurance that does not, generally speaking, include primary care services. However, because of crises and changes in their financial situations, they found themselves forced to migrate from private insurance to the public system. Thus the 'asphalt' dwellers, accustomed to the specialised services of private insurance companies, would often come to their appointments with the aim of being referred to a psychiatrist or psychologist, without expecting or desiring that a family physician evaluate or in any way attempt to treat their 'mental' needs. Among these patients, there were doubts concerning the capacity of a doctor who is not a psychiatrist to diagnose and treat mental health conditions.

For the 'hill' population, we observed that the Family Medicine physicians would more frequently use a series of consultations that they described as following a 'person-centred clinical method' (Stewart et al., 2014). These were encounters consisting of dialogues with a therapeutic goal in which the family physician would first encourage the patient to freely describe their experiences. Next, through open questions, they sought to help the patient to promote changes in their practices and behaviour that might reduce their suffering and deliver lasting improvements to their wellbeing.

The use of antidepressant medication was a common therapeutic resource among both populations, but for different reasons. According to the professionals, 'asphalt' patients demanded pharmacological treatments more frequently for two reasons. As previously stated, these patients would often seek public services because of financial downturns and, in many cases, had already begun medication treatments that had been previously prescribed by private doctors and that could not be interrupted. Additionally, in the view of the doctors, because of their 'low resilience', these patients had difficulties in overcoming depressive symptoms, even low-intensity ones, without medication. Among the 'hill' dwellers, those who sought a health service because of mental suffering did so only in severe cases, making cases of depression in the 'hill' less frequent but more severe and in greater need of pharmacological treatment.

Contact with health professionals strengthened the hypothesis that differences could be drawn between 'hill' and 'asphalt'. These involved different causes, presentations and approaches to depressive symptoms among the two populations. In order to describe these phenomena from diverse local perspectives, in addition to using the professionals' accounts, we also investigated the experiences and behaviours of the patients themselves, exploring their perceptions of their own suffering through interviews and visits to the 'hill' and 'asphalt' territories, and by following consultations. However, when studying these experiences through the perspectives of the patients, we identified limits and problems, which are described below, derived from the use of the 'hill'/'asphalt' categorisation as a way of interpreting depressive suffering of people living in a 'broken' metropolis such as Rio de Janeiro. These difficulties are illustrated by the cases of 'Raquel' and 'Pedro' (fictitious names).

'Raquel'

Raquel was a short twenty-seven-year-old black patient with close-cropped dark hair. She lived in the 'hill' and worked as a groomer at a pet store. In the first consultation we followed, she described having constant thoughts of killing herself and hearing 'voices' whose contents she was unable to identify. She lived in a small house that had two bedrooms, one for herself, the other shared by her nine-year-old daughter and sixteen-year-old son. According to Raquel herself, she had depression 'once again'. She had no desire to leave her room, where she spent most of her time alone, lying down and crying a great deal. In addition to her suicidal thoughts, Raquel recounted the need to make small cuts on her arms in order to reduce her unease when it became more intense. Among the thoughts that troubled her were her many concerns regarding her sixteen-year-old son, 'Diego', diagnosed with schizophrenia when he was ten years old, in addition to memories from a period when she lived through an aggressive marriage and the fact that she greatly missed her mother, who had passed away six months previously. She did not usually cry during consultations. Reacting to the questions posed by her physician, she alternated between looking at him and looking straight ahead while she narrated what she was feeling and thinking:

> I know I have depression and I want to get better. I know I have two children and they need me, I don't have relatives, I know I have this disease, I'm aware and I want treatment. I heard there's no cure, but there is a treatment. Depression is this sadness, like, I can't control myself when I have to cry. I just have to cry. Things don't have a solution for me. When the depression is strong, it makes you want to kill yourself. Because, like, I think death is rest. Since I lost my mother, maybe I'm like 'am I going to meet her? Or not?' But then my children are the reason for me to stay. I think if I didn't have them I would have already killed myself.

Raquel stated that she had had 'depression' crises since she was eight years old. The first episode was associated with her father's death, when she attempted suicide by taking multiple diazepam tablets. Since then, she had had similar episodes associated with specific circumstances in her life. She was divorced, but for eight years she had been trapped in a marriage in which there had been many infidelities and she had been assaulted by her husband. It took her years to leave her husband because of conflicts with her religious practices: at the time, Raquel was an Evangelical Christian. Two years previously, she had managed to leave that relationship, had stopped being an Evangelical Christian and had begun to care for her children in the house she shared with her mother.

The crisis period we followed had been triggered by her mother's death, which had taken place six months before we met her. Though some time had passed, Raquel's feelings of mourning for her mother were now intensifying. Her medical practitioner began treatment with antidepressants, in addition to an anxiolytic, clonazepam, in order to stimulate sleep until the antidepressants began to have an effect. Over the course of that same week, there were two follow-up consultations, in which the physicians was particularly concerned with evaluating the suicidal thoughts and the continued presence (or lack thereof) of the 'voices'. He also sought to promote therapeutic conversations based on a 'person-centred' approach, trying to encourage Raquel to return to activities that were good for her, such as practising jiu-jitsu.

The following week, Raquel returned for an unscheduled consultation. During the weekend, Diego had attempted sexual contact with his younger sister. Raquel became anxious and upset and did not know how to deal with this situation. She communicated the situation to Diego's father, who repeated what he had done in other situations when their son had exhibited violent behaviour: Diego was beaten as punishment for what he had done. According to Raquel, his father was the only person Diego respected, and physical aggression was the most efficient way to calm him down and make him change his behaviour. Diego was also followed by the same medical practitioner, in partnership with the 'matrix support' psychiatrist. He was medicated, but in light of this new fact, it was decided that Diego should again be referred to a Centre for Psychosocial Care (CAPS in Portuguese).[4] Though anxious and upset with Diego's situation, in that second week, Raquel reported that her depressive symptoms had already improved and that she had returned to work.

Over the course of the next three months, Raquel's 'depressive crises' occurred every three to four weeks. Taking care of Diego became harder, and she had to deal with the realisation that schizophrenia is incurable and can become more severe. Raquel was living through a confusing period, torn between whether or not she desired to have a child in her new relationship. Finally, she had been able to begin individual, biweekly psychotherapeutic sessions. The frequent consultations with the family physicians and the use of medication also continued. Of the three types of medication, she stated that clonazepam was the most helpful, both because it helped her sleep and because, according to her, it reduced her 'tensions' and 'nervousness'. She evaluated the medical care she received as very good and stated that both her physician and the 'matrix support' psychiatrist always welcomed her, talked to her at length and gave advice and guidance for Diego's care, which was sometimes better than what she received at the CAPS. In our last contact, she told us that, for the first time, Diego's father had gone to talk with the CAPS psychologist, something she believed was important because she felt that the father needed to understand Diego's problem better and to be more involved in his treatment.

'Pedro'

Pedro was a tall seventy-three-year-old white man. Born in Chile, he had lived in Brazil for over forty years. He lived in an apartment in a middle-class building in one of the main streets of the 'asphalt'. It was not a luxury building: it did not have a doorman, and the façade was old and worn. We were welcomed by Pedro and his wife, 'Laura', who was seventy years old and also Chilean. The couple were the only two residents of their apartment. When we asked what their biggest health complaints were, Pedro answered:

> What worries me most is the debts that come every month and that I can't pay entirely. My son helps me to pay them. This even affects food. Sometimes there's not enough food in our home. The standard of living we used to have is totally different from the standard of living we have now. We could go out to eat every week, we could buy new clothes, gifts for our granddaughters on their birthdays, but we can't now. All of this affects us, hurts us. Before, our granddaughters would come over on the weekend and the fridge would be full. Now, they don't come any more, because the fridge is empty. It gives me anguish,

sadness, anger, and it makes me upset. I get up in the morning and to this day I'll go take a shower thinking I'm going to work. But then it hits me.

Pedro was a retired engineer, but his income was not enough even to pay the rent. Until three years before our meeting, he had done freelance work for an important Brazilian state company. With the financial crisis that hit the state of Rio de Janeiro, these work opportunities disappeared and, even though he was retired, he found himself 'unemployed'.

One of the effects of the financial crisis that caused most suffering for Pedro and his wife was the loss of contact with their granddaughters. Their only son was in a better financial situation and frequently helped them with their expenses. However, they had problems with their daughter-in-law, who ever since they had gone into debt had, according to them, distanced herself from them and made it difficult for them to contact their two granddaughters, aged five and seven.

Pedro attributed his sadness and anger to the fact that he was unable to get work. He then stated that he was even looking for 'menial' work. However, in addition to the difficulty caused by his age, he was unable to find employment opportunities because of the serious political and economic crisis that has affected the state of Rio de Janeiro and Brazil as a whole since 2014. He also complained of weight loss. He lifted his shirt and showed us his thin body, visible bones and caved-in abdomen, stating that he had never seen himself in this condition before. He stated that he slept well but, upon waking, remembered all of his problems. He did not believe he ate poorly and claimed his appetite was normal. Because of this, he did not agree that his 'emotional state' had produced the weight loss. He was worried about his wife because he believed she was more intensely affected by their family problems than he was. He was dedicated to caring for her, even bringing her breakfast in bed every day.

Pedro had started treatment at the family health facility around two years before we interviewed him and was satisfied with the care he received from his medical practitioner. In particular, he mentioned the free examinations he had been undergoing in order to monitor his diabetes, his hypertension and a benign polyp he had in his gallbladder, in addition to the medication distributed free of charge. He wished to have an endoscopy in order to rule out a stomach ailment as a cause of his weight loss. He did not establish a clear connection between his weight loss and his 'emotional state'. To him, the 'emotional state' was connected to his 'finances'.

He was a chronic user of some other types of medication, in addition to those he used for his hypertension and diabetes. When he was 'nervous' and anguished, especially in the morning, he remembered his financial problems and took bromazepam, an anxiolytic tranquiliser, to calm down. He had always viewed himself as willing and happy to work, and he continued to feel this way. When asked whether he saw himself as having 'depression' or being depressed, he answered:

> Depression is not wanting to do anything. I was reading on the Internet, it's the person who doesn't want to do anything, doesn't want to shower, sleeps too much and has other symptoms. I don't think I have depression. My emotional state is that of unemployment, I can't pay what I owe.

In addition to his home visits, we followed two of Pedro's consultations with his medical practitioner. After checking the results of his diabetes tests, which were stable, the physician would again ask Pedro how he was feeling and he would again state his sadness, his anger at his financial situation, his concern for his wife and his thoughts of 'feeling like a nobody', especially in the mornings. The Family Medicine physician explained that depression could present itself in ways other than a desire for isolation and a lack of interest in doing anything, and that antidepressants could relieve some of those symptoms, and could perhaps even make him feel more disposed to exercise and more inclined to eat a better diet, thus helping with his weight loss. Pedro had a routine check-up, which revealed that he had no issues besides the weight loss. During this appointment, Pedro agreed to begin taking the antidepressant fluoxetine. The physician then reinforced the suggestion that he take part in some of the 'unit groups' with his wife, and he answered that it was 'a possibility'. He said he would try, but that the schedule offered was not very convenient.

Over the following months, Pedro continued to fail to gain weight, and he did not participate in any of the 'unit groups', but, after some resistance, started taking fluoxetine. However, he complained that he still saw no improvement with regard to his weight loss. He was still unhappy with his 'unemployment' and was worried about his wife. He kept regular appointments with his medical practitioner, who, in turn, insisted that he participate in the groups.

'Hill' and 'asphalt' as moral economies

Raquel and Pedro were patients considered to have depression by their Family Medicine physicians. However, the ethnographic snippets we have presented, except for the shared mentions of sadness, point to so many singularities that stating that these two people suffered from the same 'mental disorder' becomes, as Goldberg (2011: 226) noted, a form of 'magical thinking'. Even sadness, mentioned by both, was experienced differently, and these differences could not be reduced to a variation in intensity. While for Raquel it was accompanied by suicidal impulses, for Pedro it was associated with anger and motivated him to want to keep on working. The bodily manifestations – the self-mutilation in Raquel's case, and Pedro's weight loss – were also different, pointing to distinct conceptions of corporeality. In both cases, the role of micro- and macro-social determination was so evident that it is difficult to frame the situation of these individuals in terms of mental illness alone or to regard their response to these circumstances as abnormal.

Some elements of their experiences corresponded in part to the illness profiles of the 'hill' and the 'asphalt' described by health professionals. In Raquel's case, the violent interactions with her former partner, her mother's unexpected death and her difficulties in accessing adequate care in the public health system for a son with a severe mental disorder caused her suffering. In Pedro's case, social isolation, financial crisis and family problems accounted for his wife's distress. However, certain important elements did not fit this categorisation.

Raquel experienced a certain degree of isolation within her community. She had expressed a desire to move because, living in the 'hill', she still interacted with people and places that reminded her of her previous relationship, which was marked by violent situations. In the three months during which we followed her, she would again have crises marked by suicidal thoughts, isolation and self-mutilation every three to four weeks, despite a care plan that involved continuous antidepressant use, frequent consultations with her Family Medicine physician and maintaining her jiu-jitsu practice and leisure activities with her family. At the end of the observation period, Raquel attributed an experienced improvement to starting individual psychotherapy.

Pedro did not match the profile of a 'non-resilient' man that was expected from an 'asphalt' resident. He was determined to work again, if it were possible. Although experiencing low self-esteem, he reported that he was anxious to solve his financial difficulties, and did not feel sick or depressed. For this reason, he did not expect the 'unit groups' to help him with his problems, but he missed having a closer relationship with his daughter-in-law and granddaughters.

Experiences such as Raquel's and Pedro's illustrate an observation that was repeated, in different levels of intensity, with the twenty-two patients we followed more closely in the field. The classification of 'hill' and 'asphalt' that was incorporated into health professionals' discourses and practices, as well as the interpretations and clinical approaches that derive from it, did not correspond to people's experiences, and sometimes even diverged from them. On the Family Medicine physicians' side, these divergent visions of suffering have repercussions, for example, in the evaluation of many 'difficult' cases in the 'asphalt' and in the recurring statement that patients in this area do not adhere to proposed treatments, especially those in the 'unit groups'. On the patients' side, there were accounts from 'hill' patients who felt that there was a lack of specialised mental health care; this was more frequently offered to 'asphalt' dwellers, who were sometimes regarded as 'health insurance migrants' and who at times did not establish good therapeutic bonds with Family Medicine physicians.

The moral dimension of the use of social categories such as 'hill' and 'asphalt' emerged as a fundamental question for an understanding of these different diagnostic and therapeutic approaches to depressive symptoms in these settings of public integral health care. For this analysis, we turn to Didier Fassin's proposal of a critical moral anthropology as a perspective for analysing contemporary health policies (Fassin, 2008; Fassin, 2012a; Fassin, 2012b; Fassin and Rechtman, 2009), in other words, analysing how 'hill' and 'asphalt' work as 'moral economies', defined as 'norms and values, sensibilities, and emotions' that may be 'rephrased as moral', although they are not, in their usual sense, perceived to be ethical or moral (Fassin, 2012a: 4, 10).

Addressing the relationship between morals and politics, Fassin proposes that moral issues may not be understood in isolation from political, religious, economic and social spheres of human activity. One of the great enigmas in the social sciences is precisely that of the articulation between the macro-social (the different politics) and the micro-social (beliefs and practices), that is, understanding 'how public discourses and public policies influence institutional and professional practices – and are in return consolidated or sometimes reformulated through the latter' (Fassin, 2012b).

In our field of study, the explanatory model of 'lacking networks' and lacking the capacity for 'resilience' in the face of social adversities produced moral and affective approximation or distancing between physicians and patients, depending on the different population profiles. The Family Medicine physicians presented discourses and practices that were aligned with the principles of the Brazilian public health system, especially equity and the interest in offering more medical care to neglected populations, such as the 'hill' inhabitants. Some of the professionals referenced the need to overcome the 'inverse care law'. This concept was proposed in 1971 by the family physician Julian Tudor Hart, who, when analysing primary care access and therapeutic supply in south Wales, noted that the populations that least need care are the ones that have most access to health services, while the populations that most need care access these services the least (Tudor Hart, 1971; Chew-Graham et al., 2002).

The 'hill' represented a poorer population than that of the 'asphalt', less protected by social rights and policies. Nonetheless, these people were considered more resistant, with a greater sense of community and of the collective, values in tune physicians' critical views of society. On the other hand, the 'asphalt' comprised a population with better social and economic starting points, but it was more individualistic, with few community practices and values, which made it more fragile, less resistant and less willing to accept care from family physicians. Thus family physicians' social postures produced moral bonds with 'hill' patients – to whom they more frequently offered the psychosocial tools specific to their specialty, such as the 'person-centred clinical method' – and, on the other hand, a distancing from the 'asphalt' patients.

Final thoughts

In this ethnographic research, the use of the 'hill' and 'asphalt' categories as 'moral economies' has repercussions for physicians' clinical practices and patients' therapeutic experiences. The anthropological recognition and analysis of these practices provides new ways of looking at the complex social interactions that constitute the expansion of public mental health care in a Latin American metropolis such as Rio de Janeiro. It is not only 'native' medical categories, but also standardised diagnoses, protocols and treatments that produce divergences between patients and health professionals in how depressive suffering is addressed.

The acknowledgement and use of social determinants in the interpretation of, and approach to, these experiences, exemplified in this research by the categories 'hill' and 'asphalt', may also produce these dissonances, especially when we analyse their repercussions in the affections that form the terrain of therapeutic social interactions. They may also create categories that encourage 'one-size-fits-all' approaches, the focus of concerns and debate in the Global Mental Health field, as we noted at the beginning of the chapter. Sociocultural categorisations may become obstacles to more singularised evaluations of suffering, even though they are often created with the intention of producing an integral, 'bio-psychosocial' approach, as in this case study.

Therefore in this scenario, a relevant social research task is to show the role that social procedures such as the 'hill'/'asphalt' categorisation and its moral dimension have in the recognition and treatment of emotional suffering. The offer of, and justification for, biomedical resources such as psychiatric diagnoses and pharmacological treatments, and also psychosocial interventions such as 'groups' and 'person-centred consultations', were moulded by this categorisation. In this ethnographic study, we understand that making the adoption of these categories and their repercussions visible may be a useful resource for reducing barriers to understanding between health care users and professionals regarding the former's experiences of mental suffering and the latter's therapeutic practices. An important challenge for urban mental health is exploring how our experiences of the city and the environment are an important component of the construction of subjectivity, in its reflexive and emotional aspects. In a territorially 'broken' city such as Rio de Janeiro, ethnographic health research may point out paths to deconstructing often invisible social, health and moral barriers, unravelling their production processes and thus signalling the possibility of critical (re)constructions and moral proposals that, at least, reduce the weight and rigidity of social division mechanisms and the categories that derive from them.

Notes

1 There is no dataset for Rio de Janeiro comparable to the São Paulo Megacity Mental Health Survey, a population-based survey funded by WHO. The existing studies in Rio are not population-based but composed of smaller samples,

mostly from primary care services (Fortes., Villano and Lopes, 2008; Fortes et al., 2011; Gonçalves et al., 2014).
2 Over the years, part of Rio's low-income population has settled on the city's hills, forming the favelas. The city's high-income citizens usually live by the sea and in elegant planned neighbourhoods and gated communities – referred to locally as the 'asphalt' – in contrast to the hills, where urban development has little in the way of formal planning and often lacks proper infrastructure.
3 The 'matrix support' team is the Brazilian model of collaborative care in mental health within the primary care system. It involves multiprofessional teams that may include psychiatrists and psychologists. They offer 'matrix support' – a concept of work process integration in health care, developed and used in the Brazilian FHS – to assist primary care teams (Wenceslau and Ortega, 2015; Athié et al., 2016). In practice, psychiatrists consult together with the Family Medicine residents, when required by the latter. They also discuss diagnostic and treatment options with the residents.
4 CAPS are community mental health care centres that replaced psychiatric asylums following the Brazilian psychiatric reform.

References

Abas, M., Broadhead, J.C., Mbape, P., and Khumalo-Sakatukwa, G. (1994). Defeating depression in the developing world: A Zimbabwean model. *British Journal of Psychiatry*, 164(3): 293–6.

Andrade, L.H., Wang, Y.-P., Andreoni, S., Silveira, C.M., Alexandrino-Silva, C., Siu, E.R., Nishimura, R., Anthony, J.C., Gattaz, W.F., Kessler, R.C., and Viana, M.C. (2012). Mental disorders in megacities: Findings from the São Paulo Megacity Mental Health Survey, Brazil. *PLoS ONE* 7(2): e31879.

Athié, K., Lopes do Amaral Menezes, A., Machado da Silva, A., Campos, M., Delgado, P.G., Fortes, S., and Dowrick, C. (2016). Perceptions of health managers and professionals about mental health and primary care integration in Rio de Janeiro: A mixed methods study. *BMC Health Services Research*, 16, art. 532.

Caracci, G. (2006). Culture and urban mental health. *Psychiatric Times*, 23(14): 40–2.

Cavallieri, F., and Peres Lopes, G. (2008). *Índice de desenvolvimento social: Comparando as realidades micro urbanas da cidade do Rio de Janeiro*. Coleção Estudos Cariocas. Rio de Janeiro: Instituto Municipal de Urbanismo Pereira Passos.

Chew-Graham, C., Mullin, S., May, C.R., Hedley, S., and Cole, H. (2002). Managing depression in primary care: Another example of the inverse care law? *Family Practice*, 19(6): 632–7.

Chiavegatto Filho, A.D.P., Kawachi, I., Wang, Y.P., Viana, M.C., and Andrade, L.H. (2013). Does income inequality get under the skin? A multilevel analysis of depression, anxiety and mental disorders in São Paulo, Brazil. *Journal of Epidemiology & Community Health*, 67: 966–72.

Corrigan, P. (2004). How stigma interferes with mental health care. *American Psychologist*, 59(7): 614–25.

Duarte, L.F.D. (1986). *Da vida nervosa nas classes trabalhadoras urbanas*. Rio de Janeiro: Jorge Zahar Editor/CNPq.

Duarte, L.F.D. (1997). Nerves and nervousness in Brazilian urban culture. *Curare – Journal for Ethnomedicine*, 12: 21–38.

Fassin, D. (2008). The elementary forms of care: An empirical approach to ethics in a South African hospital. *Social Science and Medicine*, J67(2): 262–70.

Fassin, D. (2012a). Introduction: toward a critical moral anthropology. In D. Fassin (ed.), *A companion to moral anthropology*, 1–18. Malden: Wiley Blackwell.

Fassin, D. (2012b). Towards a critical moral anthropology: A European Research Council programme. Échos de la recherche. *La lettre de l'EHESS*, 49, http://lettre.ehess.fr/3323 (last accessed 1 November 2019).

Fassin, D., and Rechtman, R. (2009). *The empire of trauma: An inquiry into the condition of victimhood*. Princeton: Princeton University Press.

Fortes, S., Lopes, C.S., Villano, L.A.B., Campos, M.R., Gonçalves, D.A., and Mari, J. (2011). Common mental disorders in Petrópolis-RJ: A challenge to integrate mental health into primary care strategies. *Brazilian Journal of Psychiatry*, 33(2): 150–6.

Fortes, S., Villano, L.A.B. and Lopes, C.S. (2008). Nosological profile and prevalence of common mental disorders of patients seen at the Family Health Program (FHP) units in Petrópolis, Rio de Janeiro. *Brazilian Journal of Psychiatry*, 30(1): 32–7.

Galea, S., Ahern, J., Nandi, A., Tracy, M., Beard, J., and Vlahov, D. (2007). Urban neighborhood poverty and the incidence of depression in a population-based cohort study. *Annals of Epidemiology*, 17: 171–9.

Galea, S., and Vlahov, D. (2005). Urban health: evidence, challenges, and directions. *Annual Review of Public Health*, 26: 341–65.

Goldberg, D. (2011). The heterogeneity of 'major depression'. *World Psychiatry*, 10(3): 226–8.

Gonçalves, D.A., Mari, J., Bower, P., Gask, L., Dowrick, C., Tófoli, L.F., Campos, M., Portugal, F.B., Ballester, D., and Fortes, S. (2014). Brazilian multicentre study of common mental disorders in primary care: Rates and related social and demographic factors. *Cadernos de Saúde Pública*, 30(3): 623–32.

Grant, M. (2018). Planning for healthy cities. In M. Nieuwenhuijsen and H. Khreis (eds), *Integrating human health into urban and transport planning*, 221–50. Cham: Springer.

Grant, M., Coghill, N., Barton, H., and Bird, C. (2009). *Evidence review on environmental health challenges and risks in urban settings.* WHO European Centre for Environment and Health, Technical Report. WHO Collaborating Centre for Healthy Cities and Urban Policy, University of the West of England (UWE), Bristol.

Gruebner, O., Rapp, M.A., Adli, M., Kluge, U., Galea, S., and Heinz, A. (2017). Cities and mental health. *Deutsches Ärzteblatt International*, 114: 121–7.

Haroz, E.E., Ritchey, M., Bass, J., Kohrt, B., Augustinavicius, J., Michalopoulos, L., Burkey, M., and Bolton, P. (2017). How is depression experienced around the world? A systematic review of qualitative literature. *Social Science and Medicine*, 183: 151–62.

Harzeim, E. (ed.) (2013). *Reforma da atenção primária à saúde na cidade do Rio de Janeiro – Avaliação dos três anos de Clínicas da Família. Pesquisa avaliativa sobre aspectos de implantação, estrutura, processo e resultados das Clínicas da Família na cidade do Rio de Janeiro.* Porto Alegre: OPAS.

Iossifova, D., Doll, C.N.H., and Gasparatos, A. (2018). Defining the urban: Why do we need definitions? In D. Iossifova, C.N.H. Doll and A. Gasparatos, *Defining the urban: Interdisciplinary and professional perspectives*, 1–7. Abingdon and New York: Routledge.

Jenkins, J.H., Kleinman, A., and Good, B. (1991). Cross-cultural studies of depression. In J. Becker and A. Kleinman (eds), *Psychosocial aspects of depression*, 67–99. Hillsdale, NJ: Lawrence Erlbaum Associates.

Kirmayer, L.J., Gomez-Carrillo, A., and Veissière, S. (2017). Culture and depression in Global Mental Health: An ecosocial approach to the phenomenology of psychiatric disorders. *Social Science and Medicine*, 183: 163–8.

Kjellstrom, T., Friel, S., Dixon, J., Corvalan, C., Rehfuess, E., Campbell-Lendrum, D., Gore, F., and Bartram, J. (2007). Urban environmental health hazards and health equity. *Journal of Urban Health: Bulletin of the New York Academy of Medicine*, 84(3, Supplement): 186–97.

Kleinman, A. (1977). Depression, somatization and the 'new cross-cultural psychiatry'. *Social Science and Medicine*, 11(1): 3–10.

Kleinman, A., and Good, B. (eds) (1985). *Culture and depression: Studies in the anthropology and cross-cultural psychiatry of affect and disorder.* Los Angeles: University of California Press.

Krabbendam, L., and van Os, J. (2005). Schizophrenia and urbanicity: A major environmental influence – conditional on genetic risk. *Schizophrenia Bulletin*, 31: 795–9.

Lim, G.Y., Tam, W.W., Lu, Y., Ho, C.S., Zhang, M.W., and Ho, R.C. (2018). Prevalence of depression in the community from 30 countries between 1994 and 2014. *Scientific Reports*, 8(1), art. 2861.

Lopes, C.S., Hellwig, N., de Azevedo e Silva, G., and Menezes, P.R. (2016). Inequities in access to depression treatment: Results of the Brazilian

National Health Survey – PNS. *International Journal for Equity in Health*, 15, art. 154.

Macinko, J., and Harris, M.J. (2015). Brazil's family health strategy – Delivering community-based primary care in a universal health system. *New England Journal of Medicine*, 372(23): 2177–81.

Ministério da Saúde, Brazil (2012). Secretaria de Atenção à Saúde. Departamento de Atenção Básica. *Política nacional de atenção básica*. Brasília: Ministério da Saúde.

Ministério da Saúde, Brazil (2016). Departamento de Atenção Básica. Histórico de cobertura da Saúde da Família. http://dab.saude.gov.br/portaldab/historico_cobertura_sf.php (last accessed 10 May 2016).

Ministério da Saúde, Brazil (2017). Portaria nº 2.436, de 21 de setembro de 2017. Aprova a Política Nacional de Atenção Básica, estabelecendo a revisão de diretrizes para a organização da Atenção Básica, no âmbito do Sistema Único de Saúde (SUS).

Munhoz, T.N., Nunes, B.P., Wehrmeister, F.C., Santos, I.S., and Matijasevich, A. (2016). A nationwide population-based study of depression in Brazil. *Journal of Affective Disorders*, 192: 226–33.

Neri, M.C. (ed.) (2010). *Desigualdades e favelas cariocas: A cidade partida está* se integrando? Rio de Janeiro: Fundação Getulio Vargas and Centro de Políticas Sociais.

Ortega, F. (2018). 'Why not both?' Negotiating ideas about autism in Italy, Brazil, and the US. In E. Fein and C. Rios (eds), *Autism in translation: An intercultural conversation on autism spectrum conditions*, 89–106. London: Palgrave Macmillan.

Paim, J., Travassos, C., Almeida, C., Bahia, L., and Macinko, J. (2011). The Brazilian health system: History, advances, and challenges. *Lancet*, 37(9779): 1778–97.

Patel, V. (2001). Cultural factors and international epidemiology: Depression and public health. *British Medical Bulletin*, 57(1): 33–45.

Patel, V., Abas, M., Broadhead, J., Todd, C., and Reeler, A. (2001). Depression in developing countries: Lessons from Zimbabwe. *British Medical Journal*, 322(7284): 482–4.

Patel, V., and Prince, M. (2010). Global Mental Health: A new global health field comes of age. *Journal of the American Medical Association*, 303(19): 1976–7.

Patel, V., and Saxena, S. (2014). Transforming lives, enhancing communities – Innovations in Global Mental Health. *New England Journal of Medicine*, 370(6): 498–501.

Peen, J., Schoevers, R.A., Beekman, T.A., and Dekker, J. (2010). The current status of urban–rural differences in psychiatric disorders. *Acta Psychiatrica Scandinavica*, 121: 84–93.

Prado Junior, J.C. (2015). Desafios para a expansão de programas de residência em Medicina de Família e Comunidade: A experiência carioca. *Revista Brasileira de Medicina de Família e Comunidade*, 10(34): 1–9.

Rapp, M.A., Kluge, U., Penka, S., Vardar, A., Aichberger, M.C., Mundt, A.P., Schouler-Ocak, M., Mösko, M., Butler, J., Meyer-Lindenberg, A., and Heinz, A. (2015). When local poverty is more important than your income: Mental health in minorities in inner cities. *World Psychiatry*, 14: 249–50.

Silva, L., Ramalho da Silva, P.F., Gadelha, A., Clement, S., Thornicroft, G., Mari, J., and Brietzke, E. (2013). Adaptation of the Barriers to Access to Care Evaluation (BACE) scale to the Brazilian social and cultural context. *Trends in Psychiatry and Psychotherapy*, 35(4): 287–91.

Soranz, D.R. (2014). O programa de residência em medicina de família e comunidade do município do Rio de Janeiro. *Revista Brasileira de Medicina de Família e Comunidade*, 9(30): 67–71.

Steel, Z., Marnane, C., Iranpour, C., Chey, T., Jackson, J.W., Patel, V., and Silove, D. (2014). The global prevalence of common mental disorders: A systematic review and meta-analysis 1980–2013. *International Journal of Epidemiology*, 43(2): 476–93.

Stephens, C., Carrizo, A.G., and Ostadtaghizaddeh, A. (2016). Revisiting the virtuous city: Learning from the past to improve modern urban mental health. In N. Okkels, C. Blanner Kristiansen and P. Munk-Jorgensen (eds), *Mental health and illness in the city*, 465–80. Singapore: Springer.

Stewart, M., Brown, J.B., Weston, W., McWhinney, I.R., McWilliam, C.L., and Freeman, T. (2014). *Patient-centered medicine: Transforming the clinical method*. 3rd ed. New York: Radcliffe Publishing.

Thornicroft, G. (2007). Most people with mental illness are not treated. *Lancet*, 370(9590): 807–8.

Tudor Hart, J. (1971). The inverse care law. *Lancet*, 297(7696): 405–12.

Van Beljouw, I., Verhaak, P., Prins, M., Cuijpers, P., Pennix, B., and Bensing, J. (2010). Reasons and determinants for not receiving treatment for common mental disorders. *Psychiatric Services*, 61: 250–7.

van Os, J., Pedersen, C.B., and Mortensen, P.B. (2004). Confirmation of synergy between urbanicity and familial liability in the causation of psychosis. *American Journal of Psychiatry*, 161: 2312–14.

Ventura, Z. (1994). *Cidade partida*. São Paulo: Companhia das Letras.

Wahlbeck, K. (2015). Public mental health: The time is ripe for translation of evidence into practice. *World Psychiatry*, 14: 36–42.

Wenceslau, L.D., and Ortega, F. (2015). Mental health within primary health care and Global Mental Health: International perspectives and Brazilian context. *Interface – Comunicação, Saúde, Educação*, 19(55): 1121–32.

WHO (2016). *mhGAP intervention guide for mental, neurological and substance use disorders in non-specialized health settings: Mental health Gap Action Programme (mhGAP) – version 2.0*. Geneva: WHO.

WHO (2017). *Depression and other common mental disorders: Global health estimates*. Geneva: WHO.

WHO and WONCA (2008). *Integrating mental health in primary care: A global perspective*. Geneva: WHO.

WONCA (2018). Core competencies of family doctors in primary mental health care. www.globalfamilydoctor.com/site/DefaultSite/filesystem/documents/Groups/Mental%20Health/Core%20competencies%20January%202018.pdf (last accessed 1 November 2019).

8

Violence as a language of construction and deconstruction in Rio de Janeiro and Brazil

Luiz Eduardo Soares

Preface by Michael Keith

The following chapter is written by Luiz Eduardo Soares, an academic notable for a professional biography that has moved back and forth between the ivory tower and city government. Soares has served as Professor of Anthropology at the State University of Rio de Janeiro and was the National Secretary of Public Security under the mandate of Lula's presidency in Brazil.

Soares's chapter starts with the appalling statistic that between 1980 and 2010 over one million Brazilians were murdered. It is in the face of such data that violence is increasingly defined as a public health crisis in several parts of the world similarly scarred, as well as in Brazil itself. More pointedly, Soares suggests that if we are not careful such data is dehumanised. He appeals to the need to put a face to the figures. And the faces are clearly identified by the history of the city and the racialisation of the country. The faces of those who have died are massively disproportionately concentrated on one fraction of the demos of Brazil and configuration of its urban geography. As he puts it in the chapter, the victims of murder have 'a colour, a class and an address'. And in making the victims visible, in humanising the data, he argues that Rio de Janeiro can be seen as a microcosm of the country at large.

Soares has described his own paradoxical love–hate relationship with the city in the extraordinary book *Rio de Janeiro: Extreme city* (2016). The book is part autobiography of his own attempts to challenge the pandemic of violent death, and part an interdisciplinary mixture of a sociology of the city's favelas, an anthropology of the regimes of metropolitan governance and a political science of the institutional architecture of the Brazilian state. It describes in self-effacing and vivid detail his own attempts to engage, mediate, mitigate and even at times address and solve the complex system of everyday complicities between the state, its institutions and the agents of violence on both sides of the law. He describes movingly the times in which the logic of a poorly designed state architecture and the deep histories of exclusion, polarisation and racism have led to a rationally logical complicity between municipal corruption and gang violence in the favelas; how the arbitrary violence of 'pacification' of favelas masked an entrenchment rather than a solution to the powers of informally governed parts of the city where those with guns ruled. It is a story that contains both surreal humour and understated bravery.

In *Extreme city* Soares narrates how his lifetime of political engagement dating back to the fights against the military dictatorship in Brazil (1964–85) informed his links to Lula's Partido dos Trabalhadores (PT, or Workers' Party) and led him to the years of qualified optimism of urban reform in Rio. Lula's personal base always favoured São Paulo (and his football team Corinthians) over Rio, but his controversial presidency demonstrably attempted to address the scale of inequality in the country and the plight of the poorest nationally. Lula's rule overlapped with what the *Financial Times* and some economists have come to call the 'NICE' decade from 1998 to 2008. The decade was characterised by global economic growth and liberalisation of world trade with 'Non-Inflationary Continuous Expansion' the marker of most of the largest economies in the world. It also coincided with the award of the 2014 World Cup final and 2016 Olympic Games at a time when Brazil stood as one of the 'BRICS' (the B alongside Russia, India, China and South Africa). For the former Goldman Sachs guru Jim O'Neill, the BRICS were the 'rising powers' that would drive the world's economy in the twenty-first century.

So it was against this backdrop of global growth and national optimism that Soares's engagement with the governmentalities of Rio was set. His contribution to this volume links directly to Chapter 3, by McIlwaine et al., which is set in part in Maré, one of the larger favelas in Rio. In *Extreme city*, Soares describes the regimes in which the favela has for many years been under the 'drug lord control' of three factions that have operated across Rio but have divided Maré territorially between them.

Soares argued at the time for what many considered unthinkable: some kind of qualified pardoning of drug lords, linked to a peace process that learnt from international precedents. His book describes in some detail the attempts he made to realise such a change. But in the run-up to the Olympics the pressure to demonstrate the 'rule of law' across the whole of the city led to the creation of the Rio Favela Pacification Units (the UPPs). The favelas to be pacified were not chosen randomly. As he puts it, 'UPPs were established only in a few dozen locations in the Olympic belt, in other words close to wealthy neighbourhoods' (Soares, 2016: 110). As we have seen with other cities addressing the challenges of public health, Rio is driven by struggles for the future of the city shaped by its traumatic and problematic past. It is in this sense that Soares writes here against the grain of history to consider how the scars of slavery and racism underscore so many of the challenges of the contemporary moment.

For Soares the scale of violence in contemporary Brazil can be understood only through a prism of political philosophy, anthropological enquiry and forensic sociological examination of the data. It needs to be mapped against the historical legacies of the formation of the Brazilian nation state and the fusion of a Brazilian 'society' amid the legacies of treatment of indigenous peoples, the political economy of slavery and the urban realisations of colonial settlement. Soares consequently in his chapter in this volume attempts to link the philosophy of Georg Wilhelm Friedrich Hegel, the anthropology of Eduardo Viveiros de Castro and the concentrated geographies of violence to make sense of the public health pandemic that he tried to address in his time in public office in the 'extreme city' of Rio de Janeiro.

In 1807 Hegel wrote his canonical text *The phenomenology of spirit*, in which he invoked a dialectic of modernity structured by the tensions between independent and dependent self-consciousness, parsed through the relationship between master and slave. In later writing and in the Hegelian legacy in philosophy the struggle for the freedoms of self-consciousness have been cast as the master–slave dialectic. It is this dialectical relationship that forms a central theme in Soares's chapter.

Taken out of context and out of time, this becomes in Hegel's prose at worst an offensive indictment of slave consciousness, prefiguring nineteenth-century explanations of cultures of racialised poverty. So for Hegel famously 'if a man is a slave, his own will is responsible for his slavery, just as it is its will, which is responsible if a people is subjugated. Hence the wrong of slavery lies at the door, not simply of enslavers or conquerors, but of the slaves and the conquered themselves'

(Hegel, 1991, art. 57). For Susan Buck Morss (2009) Hegel has to be read historically as an author writing in the shadow of the slave rebellion that won independence for Haiti in 1804. The Haitian Revolution had exposed the border limits and hypocrisies of the French Revolution's appeal to a universal human subject. As the Caribbean scholar C.L.R. James tellingly argued in his 1938 work, Black Jacobins could make a claim in the name of *liberté*, *égalité* and *fraternité*, but slavery was to remain central to the political economy of post-revolutionary France.

More powerfully still, Paul Gilroy (1993) in his landmark postcolonial work *The Black Atlantic* argues powerfully that Hegel's master–slave dialectic should be inverted. Euro-American modernity, for Gilroy, should be viewed through lenses of the gendered subjectivities of the slave, deconstructing the myths of rational Enlightenment and its appeals to universality and progress and unpacking the colonial complicities that in part shaped contemporary liberal democracy.

In the city, just as wealth is distributed unevenly across society, so too is violence distributed unevenly across geography. These asymmetries map onto the old divisions of demos: divisions that challenge the definition of a singular 'society', pluralise a sense of publics and complicate a notion of public health in Brazil. For Soares the great migration in Brazil that increased the urban population from 37 per cent in 1950 to 86 per cent in 2010 reproduced these historical divisions in the DNA of the city. The attempt to dwell in the metropolis for those who moved, to make a home in an urban environment that was less than homely, was structured by historical racism and contemporary injustices. The chapter looks through the lens of the *longue durée* which shapes the urban form as pathogenic, the public health propensities of violence shaped by the infrastructures of twentieth-century urbanisation. Consequently, the register of voice in this chapter is very different from the discussions of public health in the rest of the volume. But the editors believe that the insights of the chapter inform and are in turn informed by an anthropological imagination that confronted the very real public health challenges of mass violence in Rio de Janeiro in recent years and provide powerful insights into the depth of deep-rooted divisions in the Brazilian city.

The end of his engagement with running national security and Rio policing was not a happy one for Soares, yet nowhere might we see better the power of the Gramscian injunction for an optimism of the soul, a pessimism of the intellect. It prompts Soares and others not to give up, perhaps matching Gramsci with Beckett's appeal to 'fail again, fail better'. It is also against the background of this biographical engagement that this chapter should be read.

Introduction

Max Weber said that the role of sociology is to exaggerate. By exaggerating, it highlights phenomena and focuses on the object. This means it is not unreasonable to draw the analogy that the city of Rio de Janeiro is a sociological version of Brazil. In other words, Carioca society, which lives in a range of different neighbourhoods and favelas, is a clear and dramatic reflection of Brazilian society itself. There are six billionaires in the country with a combined income equivalent to that earned by 50 per cent of the population – the equivalent of 105 million people; in the city of Rio, one can cross the street and go straight from areas with twenty-first-century European standards of living into some of the poorest areas in Brazil.

In the more affluent neighbourhoods of Rio de Janeiro's *Zona Sul* such as Copacabana and Lagoa, a significant proportion of the population (41 per cent and 48 per cent respectively) have a monthly income more than five times the minimum monthly wage. In favelas like Rocinha, Jacarezinho and Cidade de Deus, only 1 per cent achieve this; and in other poorer neighbourhoods like Pavuna and Santa Cruz, only 2 per cent achieve the same income (IBGE, 2010).

One of the characteristics of Brazilian society, which in Rio is paradigmatic, is the increasingly common lethal violence that has been 'naturalised' by the middle classes and the elite. The focus here is on murder. This is considered the most serious crime, and is one that leaves no doubt of its heinous violence. The historical data available goes back only to 1980; however, this data shows that such lethal violence is not 'democratically' distributed. Rather, there is a significant concentration on the process of victimisation.

The victims have a colour, a class and an address

Over the thirty years from 1980 to 2010, 1,098,675 Brazilians were the victims of murder. The figures jumped from 11.69 murders per 100,000 inhabitants in 1980 to 29.7 for the same number in 2016. In real terms, the numbers of people murdered annually increased from 13,910 to 61,158 over the whole period.

If one looks at the data for 2009, the year in which Professor Julio Jacobo Waiselfisz conducted his detailed survey, the *Mapa da violência* (*Map of violence*), published by the Ministry of Justice in 2011, one sees that 90 per cent of murder victims were male, 54 per cent were aged between nineteen and twenty-nine years, 75 per cent were killed by firearms, and 65 per cent were black. The risk of a young black male being killed is 2.96 times greater than that of a young white male. This was not an atypical year, so one can make out a pattern of deadly violence in the country that tends to affect poor disadvantaged young males, particularly black males, and that these crimes are mostly committed with guns – 76 per cent in Rio de Janeiro. It should be pointed out that this data is an accurate reflection of that for the state and city of Rio de Janeiro itself.

In 2010 the number of young people aged between eighteen and twenty-four who were in neither education nor employment in Rio was 186,133, or 26.8 per cent of the total. The highest incidences of 'neither-nor' young people were in disadvantaged neighbourhoods like Jacarezinho (38.8 per cent), Bangu (35.1 per cent) and Santa Cruz (38.4 per cent) (IBGE, 2010).

Between 2005 and 2014 there were 18,243 murders in Rio de Janeiro. The variation is more meaningful than the quantity: in 2014 murder rates per hundred thousand inhabitants in the city's most well-to-do area, the *Zona Sul*, ranged between 3.6 and 3.9, while in the *Zona Oeste* it was 34.6 and in the *Zona Norte* between 30.8 and 33.9. In addition, the three Integrated Public Safety Areas (AISPs) with the highest incidence of deaths resulting from police raids – AISP 41 and AISP 09 in the *Zona Norte*, and AISP 14 in the *Zona Oeste* – accounted for 55.5 per cent of all occurrences recorded between 2012 and 2015.

This transversal solidarity that can unite the whole city, the whole country, is rarely manifest, and appears only in the throes of indignation and cries for justice and vengeance. In general, it is reactive and negative, as fear reinforces prejudice and contributes to the intensification of inequality. In any acute crisis situation, it is natural to lean towards punitive measures. At times such as these, demagogic leaders tend to ride the tide of passion and try to connect the energy that is created with a rhetoric of greater punishment. After rebellion, the catastrophic policing and prison routines return. Nothing changes. The legal system continues to be intransigent, and the government returns to its traditional stances, with few exceptions. The Justice Department does not contemplate any change.

This gloomy scenario is not limited to the volume of murders. It also extends to the ineffectiveness of policing and investigation. According to the survey *Mapa da violência*, on average only 8 per cent of murders are actually investigated (Waisselfisz, 2011).

On the basis of this alarming information, many people assume that Brazil is a country of impunity. However, they could not be more mistaken. Brazil has the fourth largest prison population in the world. In 2013 there were already over 550,000 prisoners, whereas in the mid-1990s there were only 150,000. In 2017, although the figures have yet to be confirmed, there were a staggering 700,000 prison inmates. This increase is shocking, and its speed of growth deeply concerning.

Prisoner hunger

Of these prisoners, approximately 12,000 have been incarcerated for lethal crimes, 40 per cent of whom have yet to be formally sentenced or even gone to trial. Almost a third (28 per cent) of the prison population are serving sentences for drug dealing. It is clear that incarceration for life-threatening crime and gun use is not a priority. The focus is on drug possession and drug dealing.

In Brazil, drug dealers are expected to serve a minimum sentence of at least four years in a closed prison system, which almost completely eliminates the opportunity of any alternative penalty. Even if those who have been convicted have not been involved with gang activity, or have not committed violent crimes, they are still likely to lose their freedom. The cost to the taxpayer for each inmate is 1,500 Brazilian reales every month: a sum that could be used far more productively to transform the lives of those in prison, to promote their reintegration into society via education, employment opportunities and effective support for their families, and to offer both them and society more positive outcomes. In accordance with current legislation set by Decree 11.343/2006, drug users cannot be arrested, but should instead be taken to the local police station and then a Special Criminal Court, where they receive a verbal warning and are required to do a period of community service or a measure of compulsory attendance for an educational programme or pay a fine. Consumption of illegal drugs though continues to be considered a crime.

Brazilian law does not make a clear distinction between possession and dealing of drugs, and this further blurs interpretation by the courts and, indeed, by the police. With such blurred boundaries at their discretion, the majority of magistrates inevitably reproduce social inequalities. Their subjective assessments, which have very objective effects, tend to reiterate the discrimination of the culture in which they were brought up – one that continues to prejudice social inequality. The effects of this cocktail have been far more serious than the ingestion of any drug.

The result is the following: if the suspect is a young, white, middle-class male from a relatively affluent neighbourhood, he can defend himself with clever words: 'I'm addicted, your honour, I admit I'm a slave to addiction. But I hate having to contact dealers, I hate having to meet up with those kinds of people. I don't want to be involved with crime. That's why I buy the most I can at any one time so I don't need to meet up with them too often.' The judge usually feels sorry for the poor lad, shows clemency and doles out the treatment that he supposedly needs and deserves. In the eyes of the law, there is no doubt: *he* is a user. It will rarely occur to a similarly aged suspect who is black and poor and lives in a favela to defend themselves so cleverly. They could then run the risk of being sent down with the maximum sentence for disrespecting authority, and their explanations ridiculed. In the eyes of the law, *this* young man is a drug dealer. The middle-class white boy is seen as an 'addict', to be treated with paternalistic indulgence, while the disadvantaged black youth will be locked up for at least four years and given training for his return to freedom. Even though he may not have been violent or armed, even if he acted alone simply to make some money, he will now learn to organise himself, arm himself and use violence to achieve more ambitious aims. In Brazilian prisons, nobody survives without being affiliated to a gang.

In addition, the unfairness of the system grinds down self-esteem, and is humiliating, depressing and degrading. Prospects for escaping the cycle are minimal. This pessimistic prophecy for young offenders is almost always fulfilled, and thereby confirms prejudice, not because it is correct, but because the mediation of criminal policy transforms prediction into fact.

Police models, drug laws and the criminalisation of poverty

The steep increase in Brazil's prison population since 2003, its marked social profile and racial background, and the perverse choice of crimes that are particularly targeted are due to social and economic issues, and profound inequality and structural racism. However, although this is frequently forgotten, they are also due to the inheritance of an institutional and organisational public security structure left over from the days of the dictatorship – particularly in the way the police are organised, dividing work cycles between themselves, and in their openly militarised nature. This situation is also due to the security policies used, and it would not be possible if the disastrous approach to drug laws were not so prevalent. One should note that this institutional architecture is part of the broader field of criminal justice, and that this, in turn, means that police functioning, structured in terms dictated by a constitutionally defined model, produces dual results both with crime policies and with the connection between the civil police (non-uniformed), the Public Prosecution Office, the courts and the prison system. There is a systemic perversion of justice, with every agency sharing responsibility and being complicit in the barbarism: the prison environment is nightmarish and inhumane, and not even the state meets its own legal obligations. This brutality spills out on the streets and reconnects with its beginnings, generating and strengthening the increasingly powerful and influential criminal gangs throughout the country.

The way a group is organised is, to a greater or lesser extent, always influential in shaping the behaviour of its members: this is particularly true of institutions where discretion and arbitrary decision making are distinguished by complex, dynamic criteria and instability. In Brazil this correlation is extreme. One example is the military police, owing particularly to the nature of their duties. According to article 144 of the Federal Constitution, the military police are responsible for the public, carrying out a form of uniformed policing that is also known as preventive. Given the division of labour dictated by the same article, which assigns investigation exclusively to the civil police, the military police are responsible for undertaking arrests 'proactively', and for seizing drugs and weapons. The arrests of what kind of perpetrator, though? Acting against what kind of offence? If their duty is to get things done, and if getting things done is synonymous with making arrests yet they are not allowed to investigate, how can this problem be solved? By arresting people *in flagrante*. To what kinds of crime does this apply? There are several, but they do not include money laundering or many of the other transgressions perpetrated by white-collar criminals. The kind of people who occupy the military police prisons are almost always from the streets: pickpockets, small-time drug dealers, petty shoplifters, car thieves and so on. In general, who are the people who commit these kinds of offences? Often, they are poorly educated and disadvantaged young people from the poorer neighbourhoods and favelas, whose constant trials have led them to seek alternative routes to economic survival. The trick that makes military police action appear so 'effective' – when assessed according to rates of incarceration rather than the results that should be the priority (i.e. reducing violence) – is to make catching criminals only *in flagrante* on a widespread scale a legal tool: the criminal policy on drugs and the prohibitionist legislation from which it derives. This has created a mechanism whose smooth functioning has overcrowded prisons with young people who were unarmed when arrested, were not gang members and had not committed violent crimes. The name of this process is the criminalisation of poverty, and it is the stamp of institutionalised racism. This approach to criminal prosecution, used exclusively by the police, requires the law to be applied in a highly irregular fashion; therefore recourse to the drugs law should also fall under the remit of the basic constitutional principle of equality, class and race. It is this approach that makes access to true justice one of the most disheartening and dispiriting elements of Brazilian society. It should also be noted that the state does not meet the requirements of the criminal punishment law, and this suggests that criminals are subjected to longer incarceration than the sentences they should in fact have received. This process is particularly marked in Rio de Janeiro.

According to a survey by Luciana Boiteux (Boiteux et al., 2009), 80 per cent of those arrested for drug dealing were young people aged between sixteen and twenty-eight. Most were caught *in flagrante*, were not armed, had not committed a violent act and had no ties to criminal organisations.

State violence

There is a further element that has increased the levels of violence and requalified them. This refers, in particular, to Rio de Janeiro state between 2003 and 2016. Over this period, 12,263 people were killed through police action. The police fulfil orders and apply the lessons they learnt in training. The organisational culture has not undergone any significant revision since the dictatorship (the first fully democratic constitution was only promulgated in 1988, thus formally ending a long political transition). The enduring belief that the police are fighting a war prevails, and this means that any response is permissible. These military values define suspects as enemies to be eliminated, and define the population that lives in 'target' neighbourhoods as potential accomplices. The frequent deaths of innocent residents within poorer communities tend to be justified as accidents or as a means to an end. It is important to add that almost all the victims of extra-judicial execution are poor, young, frequently black, males from the favelas and poorer neighbourhoods.

With the development of twenty-first-century capitalism in Brazil, and perhaps because of its traditionally authoritarian background, there is a resistance to conventional social fomations, interpreted as distortions of category, experience and value. This leads to a lack of ability to nurture relationships of the 'I-You' type in the collective imagination and the day-to-day social fabric, ones that correspond to a particular kind of otherness: a kind of relational template with the 'Other' that is against violence and in favour of dialogue. This does not naively assume that in a society defined by class, and particularly in one that is so dramatically unequal, sociability can be governed by dialogue and mutual respect, thereby consecrating human rights. Brazilian society, and particularly Carioca society, stands in its structure in stark contrast to that hoped for by humanists on the basis of ethical principles and fairness. This constitutive brutality exists not only between classes or between state bodies and the less privileged classes. It is also common within the individual classes.

These tragic levels of violence have become a major reference point that both unites and separates Cariocas (in this case, the interpretation applies to Brazilian society, but they are reflected in Rio de Janeiro in a particularly significant fashion), and continue to be part of society only because of the echoes from a deeper, longer and more constitutive brutality of ontological dualism promoted by slavery and reiterated by the exploitation of labour, the magnitude of inequality, the distancing of the elitist state and the authoritarian nature of the hybrid and conservative capitalist modernisation of today's Brazil. Racism provides the historical template through which class divisions are formed in Brazilian society. Violence becomes a language, the behavioural template provided by the city to its residents, and it is within this semantic definition that the metropolis is experienced and qualified. Violence overshadows relationships and becomes second nature, undermining the republic and constructing and de-constructing identities and images of citizenship.

Historical genesis: path dependencies of slavery shaping emergent futures

The master–slave relationship is not just a few (or more) degrees more intense than any other kind of work exploitation; rather, it represents different points along a single line, or gradations along a continuum. The master–slave relationship is the ontological reduction of human beings to productive tools and commercial objects. This brutal and de-constitutive movement by the Other is unparalleled, even in the capitalist reification of workers, who are obliged to sell their labour: the two are entirely distinct processes. While from the human rights perspective people are unique and incomparable, irreducible to any equivalences and resistant to manipulation, slaves are de-personalised, de-individualised, dehumanised and reduced to a monetary series of equivalencies. The economic-political-moral-cultural operation that enslaves a human being for regular use and abuse, not only through force but also through applying an institutionalised set of standards, is a social fact, a monstrous event that introduces a second nature and creates a chasm between two ontologies.

Eduardo Viveiros de Castro's inspiring lucidity is apt here; his theory of Amerindian perspectivism inflects how we consider the dilemmas of freedom and self-consciousness and offers some enlightening analogies:

> My task was to identify elements in various indigenous cultures that would allow me to build a model that is – in a certain sense – ideal, in which the contrast with the naturalism characteristic of European modernity became more evident. … The proposition in their myths is that animals were humans but ceased to be so, and that humanity is the shared root of both humanity and animality. In our mythology, it is the opposite: we as humans were once animals, but 'ceased' to be them with the emergence of culture, etc. For us, the generic shared condition is animality: 'the whole world' is animal, but some are more animal than others, and we are the least animalistic. In indigenous mythologies, the whole world is human, only some are less human than others. There are several animals that are very distant from human beings, but they are all, or almost all, human in origin, and this goes against the idea of animism, which is that the universal foundation of reality is the spirit. (Viveiros de Castro, 2008: 480)[1]

The myth for the origins of Brazilian society tells the story of three races that formed a fellowship, combining their strengths to form the

Brazilian nation: native Indians, Africans and white Europeans. The European colonisation of Brazil tells a different story, in which the native Indians and the Africans were taken advantage of to build the power and wealth of the white Europeans, themselves divided between the exploited and the exploiters. What is important to focus on here is the introduction of a different symbolic constellation, the roots of which were sown deep in the experiences of individuals and which marked all social relationships. The slaves were not humans who had been animalised in order to become goods and tools of labour; neither were they animals that had reached a subhuman intermediary stage to serve their masters, with the hope of perhaps one day achieving full human status. Slavery instils a third ontological order, for which both descriptions are inappropriate. This ontological displacement is in the perspective of the masters, the law and the institutions, and is manifested in the field of social practices. Slavery is exile from humanity. Resistance does not come only through direct confrontation. It also comes from the silent insistence of knowing oneself to be human, and from asserting one's sense of dignity despite the white exploiters' attempts to destroy this. Even if they do succumb to their master's humiliating orders, slaves cannot be criticised or judged, as they are merely accepting what liberal countries called the 'natural law' in order to survive (Pinsky, 2010). This means that slavery did not actually degrade slaves' humanity, as they were the victims. Rather, it degraded that of the masters and exposed their moral turpitude from the perspective of those whom they exploited: the slaves. However, from the perspective of the masters, the slaves were nothing more than goods. Two dehumanities lived alongside each other but could not relate – one produced by the violence of slavery and the commercialisation of human beings, and the other produced for the benefit of the masters, their sidekicks and those who stood to benefit from the system. Slavery is not a relationship. The two ways of being show an ontological duplicity.

The hypothesis of a dual ontology

There is no communication between the two ontologies: slaves do not suddenly become human to their masters when they are caressed, or when their human attributes – sexual and emotional – are recognised. They may be treated with kindness, but they continue to be slaves, remaining within the inhuman order to which they belong – inhuman from the point of view of practice, abiding laws, the economy that needs them and the exercise of power. There is no oscillation between being and not being a slave according to a master's moods and desires or depending on the communicative register or the way the patriarch chooses to treat his slaves. The erotic idyll of a loving partner cannot be such for a libidinous master, as because she is a slave, the woman is dehumanised; she cannot ever be the equal of the master. She is only an object, no matter how she temporarily experiences the transference of herself to a second body that corresponds to the human soul. In this case, the double of the slave woman exists only as that seen by the master, even though his lover may occasionally play the game and confirm the reality of the meeting and become displaced emotionally and notionally. It is a vicarious topology – one that is subject to the master's emotions, and it does not imply any recognition of the human nature of the Other, the woman who is desired. The real woman under the guise of a slave is a real human being, a subject, and is somewhere else, beyond the master's reach, his power, his values and his logic. The second body of the slave is reduced to a fantasy phallocentric projection and the extension of patriarchal authority, even though the woman who is coveted may provisionally identify with this second body and inhabit it in a similar way to a visitor to a theme park. From the most extreme slavocratic hypothesis – and from the perspective of the organisation of social power, morality and the ontological reduction of otherness – there is no difference between using the Other for pleasure or suffering if the choice comes from one's own desire, and the Other has no choice but to fulfil their designated role. This means that there is no difference if the Other is excluded from the inter-subjective dynamics in which they would hold the role of the subject – and it is this that is so important in any recognition of their humanity.

A slave cannot be a 'you' for an 'I' master in an idealised dialogue, because their position is reified as that of a third party. Direct communication flows through the rules of a machine-like, consequential and non-dialogical pragmatism: orders are transmitted and their targets are receptors; it is inappropriate to speak unless it is in order to clarify the order received – which is part of the expectations. This form of communication differs from that practised in hierarchically organised institutions, as in these it is the positions and not the individuals that make speech function as orders. In an institutional context, positions are held by individuals whose authority is reversible and conditioned. Contrastingly, the word 'slave' is the name of a position that is then transformed into a quality of 'person' without anything else. The designation of 'slave' strips away humanity because the word itself (and of the institution that represents it) promotes simplification, reducing it to its representation in the logic of power. If the name mirrors the thing, it is because pragmatically it constitutes it by creating a result through the act of speaking. This result neutralises potential virtues, indeed, it neutralises itself, because in this case destiny does not involve unpredictability or a random game of chance. The definition of a slave defines a being and remains frozen in time. Slaves can be bought and sold, taken from one town to another, from one workplace to another, can provide sexual services to their masters – but they cannot be what they are not. While they are alive, they will always be slaves. In this sense, they have no past or future, and not even their children are their own.

What really happens when the veto on inter-subjectivity is imposed and thus cancels out any possibility of dialogue? One answer can be found in Eduardo Viveiros de Castro's interpretation of another impossible dialogue:

> Following the analogy with the pronominal series (Benveniste 1966a, b), one can see that, between the reflective *self* of culture (the generator of the concept of the soul or spirit) and the impersonal *it* of nature (a marker of the relation to otherness), there is a discursive position of the *you*, the *second person*; of the *other* considered as another subject, whose point of view serves as a latent echo of the *I*.
>
> I believe that this concept can help one to determine the supernatural context. It is an abnormal context in which the subject is seen from another dominant cosmological point of view, where it is seen as the *you* from a non-human perspective; *the supernatural is the form of the Other as the Subject*, implying the objectification of the human 'I' as a you for this Other.
>
> The typical supernatural situation of the Amerindian world is the encounter in the forest between a human being – always alone – and a being that, *seen* primarily as a mere animal or person, reveals itself as a spirit or a ghost, and *speaks* with the man.... These meetings are often lethal for the interlocutor, who, subjugated by his non-human subjectivity, passes to the other side, becoming transformed into a being of the same species as the locutor: whether dead, spirit or animal. Those who respond to a *you* spoken by a non-human accept the condition of being their 'second person', and thereby accepting the position that *I* will have as a non-human.... Thus, the canonical form of these supernatural encounters consists in the sudden insight that the other is human, that *he*

is human, and this automatically dehumanises and alienates the interlocutor, transforming them into prey – into an animal. This is the true significance of the Amerindian disquiet about what lurks beneath appearances. Appearances can be deceptive, as one can never be sure about what is the dominant point of view, or rather, of which world is interacting with the Other. Everything is dangerous; especially when everything is human, and perhaps, we are not. (Viveiros de Castro, 2008: 396–97; author's italics)[2]

This is a long quotation, but it sheds such light on the question that I feel readers will forgive me. By applying this analysis to the slavocratic cosmos at the points where the analogy seems relevant, and returning to the initial argument, one can conclude the following: if the master personalises the slave, and the latter, recognising their own humanity (recognising themselves as *the* human), takes part in this dialogical game and accepts the place of 'secondary person' to the master, they will lose their humanity and their autonomy, because they have allowed the master's point of view to prevail and have thereby validated the corresponding world, a world in which they are slaves, objects, prey, tools, property, things and beasts of burden. This makes it lethal for slaves to take a generous, compassionate and empathic approach, or to try to understand the master as anOther human being, hiding their own nature under the iniquitous arrogance of ownership. It is deadly because it subtracts from humanity, and returns it to the third nature – that of slavery.

Avoiding or hiding from dialogues with the master (which in themselves are a trap because inter-subjectivity is impractical in this case), putting them off or trying to adopt evasive or confrontational strategies are all manifestations of resistance and of struggling for freedom and autonomy: they are the preservation of humanity itself. These manifestations should not be construed as an expression of hatred or resentment, as what is at stake is the threat of abducting slaves' humanity.

The lethal risk of succumbing to the master's seduction and moving into the space of the *second person* is unconsciously assimilated, and therein transmutes into the chronic and omnipresent suspicion that contaminates the culture for future generations and that may for some – even if widely justified – eventually appear to be a kind of paranoid atavism resistant to cooperation and contract and sceptical of politics and justice. This persistent suspicion is particularly harmful and damaging as it concerns not only the Other, but also the *self* through the mediation of the Other: if the world in effect denies even the descendants of slaves their humanity because of the continued presence of racism and extreme inequality, identifying with it, belonging to it and sharing its nature may lead to the discovery of a shared inhumanity. In the words of Viveiros de Castro, quoted above, on a structurally analogous situation: 'Everything is dangerous; especially when everything is human, and perhaps, we are not.'

Colour as the language of inequality and class

I have tried to set out the reasons for rejecting any balance between antagonisms when describing the experience of slavery in Brazil. Applied to this specific historical context, ontological discontinuity contests concepts of permeability, hybridism and the juxtaposition of opposites and ambiguity. In this sense, I see Brazil as the reverse of the way in which it is usually described. Racism is not a manifestation of prejudice dislocated from the poor or less advantaged classes. It is quite the opposite: racism came first, and is manifest through its effect of dislocation. The root of the problem is the institutional lacuna in republican modernity that translates into a non-tacit prejudice against black and indigenous peoples, and into resisting any recognition (and experience) of individuality in a contemporary sense. It seems to me that Brazilian society is centred on great inequality, and that this ontological dualism normalises and polarises ordinary inequalities. It is as if the ontological duality that no longer exists is still vibrating and shining like stars that have been dead for millennia, and is still able to illuminate paths through the night. The light of these extinct stars continues to warp the refracted social perception through a game of smoke and mirrors, and we continue to be deceived by it and to reify it, forgetting its origins and emulating the characters of the platonic caveman myth.

The ontological duplicity instilled by slavery did not cease to exist with the legal end to slavery in 1888: the effects on Brazilian society remain as deep scars, or tattoos, and the effects have not disappeared with the mere passage of time. The marks do not disappear as they are gradually forgotten, because new experiences replace previous ones. Given the long-lasting significance of slavery and the pain involved, forgetting, denying or underestimating its importance will only transform the tragedy into trauma. All the repressed suffering comes back but in a different place, resistant to interpretations, haunting, disturbing and disseminating feelings of fear, insecurity and hate. Rather than easing the suffering and memory of the horrors, the absence of wider societal recognition of what slavery meant to the native Indians and African Brazilians on a national scale actually perpetuates the pain and distances it from its roots. The celebration of a mixed-race, syncretic Brazil has been positive, but it has also had a heavy toll on many. This is because the valuation of a mixed-race Brazil has not come about as a clear response to the horrors that were perpetrated, which would involve public commitments to reverse the inequalities to which black people continued to be condemned even after abolition. It is true that miscegenation has defeated the hegemony of racism in a sense; however, it has done so by accentuating the contiguous line of the colonial past. Freirean theory, which it legitimised, mitigated the oppression of slavery, as if the justification of any positive reading of the miscegenation of races depended on establishing a bond with an underlying trend that was already, in its embryonic form, detectable at the heart of slavery. Miscegenation was the natural progression of Portuguese flexibility transplanted to the tropics. In other words, it would be a later stage of Brazilian historical evolution that would update aspects already present in the previous stages, giving them continuity over any negative, brutal and uncivilised elements. Brazilian wisdom would be able to dispose of negative components, and conserve power for the worthy.

Miscegenation would decant slavery, and thereby transcend it. This narrative does not account for the monster. It does not elaborate on the horror, or pronounce its name. Neither does it process – symbolically, emotionally or intellectually – the rupture that has happened culturally, if not politically. To name the horror, to recognise it, means marking a cut and a passage, means giving it meaning, circumscribing it and creating the conditions to overcome it, absorb it and battle it. The act of saying implies the act of doing, as the narratives in this case are also performative. We make things with words. The democracy of uniting the races until this nefarious concept becomes extinct is a beautiful ideal, but not if it happens through an origin myth that censures the horror, through the fairy-tale that racism does not exist in Brazil, or through the argument (which, while I realise it is well-intentioned, is in my opinion mistaken) that talking about it, denouncing it and applying policies to mitigate its effects are ways to involuntarily produce or strengthen it.

This ontological duality loses institutional rooting, and slips down an economic platform open to mediations that encourage the conversion of slave-property into an intensely exploited work force-commodity, in environments that lack economic, social, civil and political rights, and that are marked by the predominance of racist, authoritarian and hierarchical (whether patrimonial or class-led) cultural formations. One should remember that (limited) labour guarantees were applied only in the 1960s – and came at the same time as the political repression imposed by the dictatorship and by oligarchic violence.

Seen in this context, the great migration corresponded to a displacement of tectonic plates, deepening inequality and producing further traumatic experiences.

The great migration

From 1950, and particularly from the start of the period of accelerated industrialisation in the middle of the decade until the end of the 1970s, it is estimated that 35.4 million people migrated from rural areas of Brazil to the cities. In 1950 only 36.63 per cent of the Brazilian population lived in cities. By 1980 the morphological configuration of traditional Brazil was reversed: 70.32 per cent of the population was urban. In 2010 86.11 per cent of the Brazilian population lived in cities. In view of the size of the population and the speed of change, especially between 1950 and 1980, the phenomenon was extraordinary. It should also be noted that, at its peak, this process took place under the dictatorship. These migrants did not have any channels of expression of their own, any tools of organisation, nor could they count on any welfare state worthy of the name. They were launched into the urban jungle in their millions.

The effects were traumatic and the factors of migration, which were in general negative, showed that the attractions and opportunities offered by industrial modernisation were outweighed by the hardships encountered by workers, who found themselves subjected to ruthless exploitation. 'The forced displacement to the cities ... was, in the great majority of cases, experienced as a process of loss and decay', in the words of Moacir Palmeira and Afrânio Garcia, whose work in this area has been very important (Palmeira and Garcia, 2001: 65).

Without a doubt, it would be a mistake to generalise such varied emotions and personal and collective experiences: indignation at the poverty, humiliation and abuses; hopes for a better life; fear of the unknown; and worry. These were then followed by the stresses of arriving and the need to search for a place to live and work. In many cases, the original networks from the rural community were restructured in the city, at least partially. Those who arrived first and managed to settle themselves acted as the trailblazers, paving the way for family, friends and neighbours: they gave advice, shelter, guidance, mediation and help. Others arrived on the off chance, unprepared, sleeping anywhere, eating whatever they could find, taking any opportunity offered. Between these two oppositional narratives is a multitude of others. There was no single path or destination. There was a vast range of adaptive dynamics, depending on the context and individuals' ability to weave personal relationships or find occupations that would guarantee survival.

Despite these considerations about the errors of generalisation, it is reasonable to assume that there are some shared characteristics. Either at the same time or in stages, fathers, sons, mothers and entire families made the exodus from the countryside to the cities – which were not ready or willing to offer shelter, and the crystal broke into a thousand pieces. They ended up having to build shacks that were merely premature ruins. They aged prematurely, under the extreme pressure from such radical change. The effort to adapt is not simple. It would be wrong to think of the adaptive process by seeing the subject from the perspective of two different objects: the prior fully coded life, and then the urban life waiting to be mapped out; all that are needed are a cognitive process, and the simple exchange of a hoe for a cement wheelbarrow. If it were this simple, migration would be merely a combination of learning and willpower: all that migrants need to do is change their belief systems so that their new lives in the city will match new categories. This analytical way of thinking is incorrect. It misses out something essential – which is that, in addition to the brutality of the impoverishment of this process, the people who suffer the most radical impact are the subjects themselves. They are not the same in the two scenarios. It is true that the objects change, but the subjects are not static either. They literally lose their ground. It was not their knowledge that told them what their lives were before the exodus; it was their lives before the exodus that told them who they were. This previous life was composed of many ingredients: the community, family, work, the land, the landscape, belief systems, values, the temporality of rural life, and the rhythms and upsets of nature.

It is true that rural life is not always a harmonious community experience between peers, fellow workers and their families – not to mention the oppressive relations with those who are unequal, because these are ubiquitous. In the extreme and tragic case of drought driving away the people of the land, the social fabric becomes frayed. In the Brazilian reality, it is worth repeating that the routes to migration have been multiple. There are many migrants who have managed to overcome hardships and challenges and redefine their crossing over as liberation. Lula, Luiz Inácio Lula da Silva, was a migrant who became president and a national hero, and became an icon of affluence at all levels.

The radicalism of change

One can learn from Tim Ingold – and numerous Brazilian writers and poets – that human beings do not live in a single place. We cannot even say that we are part of a place, as we are, in part, the place itself. Admitting this is tantamount to acknowledging that migration on a wide scale corresponds to a displacement of the tectonic plates of Brazilian society. This event will continue to have long-lasting repercussions. To a certain extent, the men and women who migrated travelled far from *themselves*, distanced themselves from who they were, and perhaps even lost themselves. In the city, they threw themselves into the radical adventure of inventing a new subject, a new character for themselves, a person they could inhabit, someone who inhabited the city, a place entirely strange – the strangeness being intensified through involving both the relations of the subjects to themselves and the subjects' relations with their new social universe, new language and new way of life.

Tim Ingold is the anthropologist who has perhaps written most extensively and profoundly on this. In contrast to the Western supremacy of form over process, he posits the 'dwelling perspective' as opposed to the 'building perspective' (Ingold, 2000: 173). Reflecting on the Heideggerian idea that there is a significant difference between dwelling and living and between a house and a home, Ingold believes that there is much more in the experience of living than simple occupation. Living goes beyond the separation between public and private; it transcends the limits of a domestic home and extends its content to being in the world: 'thus "I dwell, you dwell" is identical to "I am, you are"' (Ingold, 2000: 185).

In addition to the category 'dwell', Ingold works with the concepts of landscape and temporality, distinguishing them from those of land and chronology: 'where land is thus quantitative and homogeneous, the landscape is qualitative and heterogeneous' (Ingold, 2000: 190). Landscape is not to be confused with the concepts of nature and space, and neither should temporality be diluted through calculable extension and isomorphically divisible units of physical time. Temporality is the social journey of human beings through the landscape, marking it with the dynamic experience of living through the cycle of life; dwelling is understood as being in the landscape, engaged in it through all kinds of activities and interactions, each of which corresponds to different paths. He teaches us that every map is encapsulated in a way of life (Ingold, 2000: 225).

Ingold shows that the analytical separation between a tradition and its territory, and between a culture and its place, means becoming distanced from the traditional knowledge of the context in which it was produced, and from the practical experience from which it emerged. This is experience situated in a specific and ecologically significant environment. The consequence of this artificial separation is to reduce a 'form of life' to a 'world view' or 'cognitive schema' (Ingold, 2000: 225). This intellectual movement is like the transposition of an organic immersion, from the phenomenological perspective, to the metaphysics of representation that operates through the dualism of subject–object.[3]

If one agrees with Ingold and applies his perspective to the great migration in Brazil, this presents new challenges. To reiterate, as perhaps now the argument has become clearer: this vast migration can be compared to a dislocation of the tectonic plates of Brazilian society. It was the subjects themselves who suffered the most radical impact of this transformation process, as they could not be the same in both settings. Objects change, settings change, and the subjects change too. They literally lose their ground. To reiterate: it was not their knowledge that told them what their lives were before the exodus; it was their lives before the exodus that told them who they were. The echo of ontological duality is reclassified but remains undiluted. On the contrary, if becomes more concentrated.

Democratic transition detached from the masses

There is another key point here: it was in this context that the transition to democracy was enshrined in the promulgation of the Federal Constitution in 1988. This coinciding of two such different temporalities, the great migration and the change of regime, may help to explain the distance between the civic enthusiasm of Ulysses Guimarães (a federal deputy, and then president of the Chamber of Deputies), holding up the new constitution, the new social contract – the sign of his triumph in the National Congress – and the indifference of the people, with an ingrained scepticism of a system that encouraged inequality and the continuation of societal injustice. On one hand there was the institutional language of the state, and on the other there were the still audible echoes of ancestral ontological dualism, the delayed eloquent vibrations of the unsaid and the persistence of historical traumatic repression.

More than three decades have passed since the democratic state of law was established. More than thirty years of advances, macro-economic stabilisation, poverty reduction, expansion of citizenship, cyclical electoral mandates – this is what one would have said before the huge crisis that has engulfed the country since 2015. And despite the advances (which are now being challenged if not revoked), relations between state and society are still marked by mistrust and tutelage; and, with the crisis, this is only increasing. The inequality of access to justice continues to resist change, and the mechanisms that reproduce the order still perpetuate the atavistic face of police brutality against blacks and the vulnerable poor. Unfairness, violence, environmental destruction and representational crisis coexist alongside more widely celebrated achievements. In this wave of inert reiterations, the trail of ontological dualism rips the surface of society like a scar resistant to change, avoiding the official maps.

Synthetic conclusions

The above leads one to the following hypotheses.

(1) The ontological duality initiated by four centuries of slavery, which has continued through the racism and injustice in the twentieth century and been repressed in the national memory, finds creative and reversive approaches when the cultural and social dynamics of the 'I–You' type erupt, radically transforming the process of circulating voices, lines of power and authority, and deposits and sources of value. For example, Tropicalism was (and has left us with) an experimental laboratory for a new 'I–You' individuality and dialogue.

(2) The dialogical scheme in the relationship with alterity cannot be consolidated without socio-economic transformations and radical policies, and without reducing inequalities and addressing structural racism in all its manifestations.

(3) Any acceptance in Brazilian society of a new model of relating to the Other involves, implies and presupposes the establishment of

interventions (always multidimensional) aimed at building and maturing individuality, as subjective and inter-subjective experience, as a judicial-political category in the field of rights and as the source and target of values – the basic meaning of which is dignity. To this end, the combined yet unequal development of capitalism, even with its authoritarian nature, has paradoxically – or dialectically – contributed to and generated our conservative modernisation. This has happened because the paroxysmal progression of individualism, so desired by globalised market dynamics, generates a further contradiction by creating conditions in which individuals can go through the looking glass, radicalise their experiences and escape the commercial orbit that defines them as consumers and reduces them to mere calculations of utility and function.[4] This liberating process requires an insidious and capillary revolution, one that has potential to reach a historic scale.

(4) Outside parties and institutions, and in the midst of so many tensions, individuality starts to grow in Brazilian society, an individuality that is constructed, lived, strengthened and expanded by social groups and individuals for whom the axis of accretion is on a plane that is invisible to anyone who sees only conjuncture or focuses on traditional sociological variables, which separate reality into layers. The strength of individuality and of the individuals and groups who embrace it creatively, in its multiple dimensions, cannot be identified or evaluated by sectoral analyses that look at human rights, values and subjectivities, and to a lesser extent, the market or the world of institutional interests and policies, even though all these areas are pertinent and relevant. There has been more space (even though any generalisation is of course overly simplistic and incorrect) to respect the individuals who dare to reinvent themselves from their own personal grammars, who rebel against labels and classifications, diagnostics and stigmas, fixed judgements and the determination of biographical fate, without cutting ties with their experience of empathy and solidarity, and recognising the same freeing potential in the Other. Meandering and highly individualised itineraries in religion, or in the field of spirituality, are just one example among many that bear witness to this trend. Experiments that distinguish body, sex, gender and identity also represent cutting-edge contributions that are of great importance for individuality. In the midst of intolerant reactions, and often with great difficulty, these inventors of themselves (in connection with collective agenda and repertoires) have achieved remarkable successes in the country, broadening the territory of individuality as

experience, and pointing to correspondent reconstruction whether in the sphere of category, of the law or of value, promoting the substitution of morality as a code for that of morality as openness to the Other and availability. Minority movements with connections to the defence of religious tolerance and liberty play a decisive role. Even though they are not strictly minorities, the feminist and anti-racist movements are stronger and better nourished by these virtuous dynamics, and this opens space in the midst of so many different barriers and forms of social, economic and cultural oppression.

(5) In addition, in parallel to the modest but significant reduction of poverty, for two decades the country has seen an increasing valuation of equality and the language of citizenship – running the risk, it is true, of the reductionist judicialisation that drains policies and invades privacy. However, going in the opposite direction of this democratising process is the counter-reformation, guided by a neo-liberal economic governance agenda in alliance with the most conservative moral supporters and skilled at articulating themselves with rhetoric, calling for tougher laws, longer sentences, more freedom for the arms trade, the war against drugs and the criminalisation of poverty, and more police violence. To crown this perverse agenda, they advocate policies that destroy the environment and annihilate the lands of the indigenous peoples. Under such an empire of hatred, the political culture is impoverished and retreats, blunting the imagination and dialogue, which ends up being fairly consistent with the role accorded to Brazil by the international division of labour. The country seems resigned to its agro-exporter fate, even in the twenty-first century.

One must conclude by admitting that, despite the fine words and the glimmer of other hopeful possibilities, the remains of this ontological duality are still among us, ripping at the heart of the country. Hatred has not ceased to circulate in the veins of the sleeping giant. It flows like a river of blood whose source has never ceased to be the masters' house.

And that is Rio de Janeiro.

Notes

1 Translations in this chapter were commissioned by the editors of the volume except where otherwise stated.

2 Translated from the Portuguese translation of the original French source text.
3 It is interesting here to compare Ingold's position to the pragmatism of William James (2000) and Richard Rorty (1979), in whose works – other than specific differences – the disposal of the Cartesian pair does not give rise to a holistic concept, but rather to a dislocation of *cogito* to *praxis*, which brings Ingold back into the conversation.
4 For the analysis of a further seventeen contradictions, see David Harvey (2016).

References

Benveniste, É. (1966a). De la subjectivité dans le langage. In Benveniste, É., *Problèmes de linguistique générale*, 258–66. Paris: Gallimard.
Benveniste, É. (1966b). La nature des pronoms. In É. Benveniste, *Problèmes de linguistique générale*, 267–76. Paris: Gallimard.
Boiteux, L., Wiecko, E., Batista, V.O., and Prado, G. M. (2009). Tráfico e Constituição: Um estudo sobre a atuação da justiça criminal do Rio de Janeiro e de Brasília no crime de tráfico de drogas. *Revista Jurídica*, 11: 1–29.
Buck-Morss, S. (2009) *Hegel, Haiti and universal history*. Pittsburgh: University of Pittsburgh Press.
Gilroy, P. (1993). *The Black Atlantic: Modernity and double consciousness*. Cambridge, MA: Harvard University Press.
Harvey, D. (2016). *17 contradições e o fim do capitalismo*. São Paulo: Boitempo.
Hegel, G.W.F. (1991). *The elements of the philosophy of right*, trans. H.B. Nisbet, ed. A. Wood. Cambridge: Cambridge University Press.
Hegel, G.W.F. (2018). *The phenomenology of spirit*, trans. M. Inwood. Oxford: Oxford University Press.
IBGE (Brazilian Institute of Geography and Statistics) (2010). *Censo 2010*, https://censo2010.ibge.gov.br/en/noticias-censo.html (last accessed 1 November 2019).
Ingold, T. (2000). *The perception of environment: Essays on livelihood, dwelling, and skill*. London: Routledge. Kindle ed.
James, C.L.R. (1938). *The black Jacobins: Toussaint l'Ouverture and the San Domingo Revolution*. Harmondsworth: Penguin.
James, W. (2000). *Pragmatism and other writings*. New York: Penguin.
Palmeira, M., and Garcia, A. (2001). Transformação agrária. In I. Sachs, J. Wilhelm and P.S. Pinheiro (eds), *Brasil, um século de transformações*, 38–77. São Paulo: Companhia das Letras.
Pinsky, J. (2010). *Escravidão no Brasil*. São Paulo: Editora Contexto. Kindle ed.
Rorty, R. (1979). *Philosophy and the mirror of nature*. Princeton: Princeton University Press.

Soares, L.E. (2016). *Rio de Janeiro: Extreme city*. London: Penguin.
Viveiros de Castro, E. (2008). *A inconstância da alma selvagem*. São Paulo: Cosac & Naif.
Waiselfisz, J.J. (2011). *Mapa da violência*. Brasília: Ministério da Justiça.

9

Conclusion: city DNA, public health and a new urban imaginary

Michael Keith and Andreza Aruska de Souza Santos

In the introduction to this volume we argued that the new data-rich urban sciences generated a power to read the city differently when making sense of the interface of public health and metropolitan systems. The potential of new forms of measuring, quantifying and interrogating behaviour at scales that can move from the demos to the individual and back again is immense. But this does not imply a straightforward celebration of cities that are putatively 'smart' or public health systems that are straightforwardly technocratically driven. We know that powers of prediction are qualified by the (in)stability of the systems – or systems of systems – in which they are rooted. Health systems are particularly subject to rapid and disruptive technological change, contested ethical settlement and imperatives to optimise prevention and treatment of different pathologies through competing systemic measures of valuation of public goods and private rights and obligations.

We also suggested that an appeal to 'public' health is implicitly an invocation of the city as commons, the urban figured as a space in which public interests might trump individual rights. It is also a space in which time is embedded in geographical practice (as Schwanen and Nixon discuss in Chapter 4). Public health systems always balance what is plausible in the immediate present with what might be possible in the near and distant future. These sorts of trade-off and the instabilities of complex systems are as true in cities of the global south as they are in the global north. In this sense health features prominently in 'development policy' in the cities of the global south that constitute an increasingly significant proportion of planetary urban life. There is also an unpardonable neglect of the scholarship of the global south in mainstream urban studies in social science. But there is in truth much that might be learnt between cities across both sides of the global north–south divide – but only to an extent.

In urban hierarchies that are frequently structured by past and present forms of intense polarisation and exclusion, and in countries that see massively varied levels of life expectancy within cities as much as between them, the importance of understanding context needs to be read alongside the sometimes limited potential to shape city futures differently. The path dependencies and lock-ins of different urban systems undermine a sense that there are invariably universal 'solutions' to generic 'problems'. What works at one scale might not work at another. The pressing demands of the present and the imperatives to intervene in settings of gross injustice or times and places of 'emergency' in the present day might properly prioritise 'clumsy' or pragmatic solutions over elegant and systemic optima.

In framing the city through the lens of public health there is always a risk that a critique of certain universalising narratives of urban change rejects crude generalisation in a plaintive but ultimately banal appeal to the unique character of each and every different urban settlement. However, such an appeal falls into the trap of seeing both time and space as merely measurements of distance and chronology. In contrast we would prefer a sense of a more dynamic characterisation of both the historicity of the temporal and the spatiality of the geographical situated within the relational patterns of global urban transformation. We have argued in this volume that this trap can be avoided by situating the particular within a complex systems framing that both surfaces the ethical choices that have structured the inequalities of the city and makes sense of the universal in the context of the path dependencies of the active and disruptive historicities and spatialities of the metropolis. So, for example, in this volume Wenceslau and Ortega foreground the geographies of the Brazilian city in structuring the propensities of mental health (Chapter 7), and Soares its racist history (Chapter 8). And so 'knowing the future city' demands an ability to jump between scales and time frames; to think locally and act globally; to look backwards to make sense of what is to come.

Several of the chapters in this volume, such as those by Rose (Chapter 2), McIlwaine et al. (Chapter 3) and Schwanen and Nixon (Chapter 4) link cities of the global north and the global south – at some times through the cultural traffic of international flows of people and ideas, and other times through a sense of the comparative. There is a long and at times problematic history of comparative studies in the social sciences, but for the purposes of this volume it is perhaps most important to emphasise how different chapters make visible similar logics in rapidly changing empirical contexts. The emergence of four decades of exponential growth in China since Deng's 'opening up' qualifies any suggestion that the country's urban transformation constitutes a form of urbanism of the global south. The 'modernisation' of cities in Brazil and South Africa qualifies the extent to which urban transformation can be seen straightforwardly through a lens of 'development'. Some motifs run through the past and return in histories of the present city across the globe.

For example, in this volume's chapter on food security, the rational push towards land-use zoning and the creative responses of the informal (Smit) are partly structured by appeals to good governance. And while effective urban planning and management undoubtedly play a central role, the appeals to rationalise the city have been problematic throughout the history of the urban. The rational city is an object that sits on the horizon of the urban, frequently just beyond the field of vision of the people who live in cities. It invokes an aspiration that is one of 'development' today in Lagos and London alike. The technocratic appeals to mobility and public health wellbeing seen in Rio and London today (Schwanen and Nixon in Chapter 4), food security and land-use zoning in Africa (Smit in Chapter 6), or sensible sanitation in China (Iossifova in Chapter 5) all in part share a sense of the city as a modernist mirage. The city can be rationalised 'if only', for as Bruno Latour famously said, 'we have never been modern'. To steal a phrase, we might almost say that 'we have never been urban'; the good city is an ideal type that collides with the reality of path dependency and lock-in, at times confounding the logics of technocratic solutions to independently defined problems.

So what we are arguing for in this volume is an urban imaginary that learns geographically but is sensitive historically and recognises that generalisable behavioural trends globally need to be reconciled with the logics of cities whose DNA may differ very widely. Just as the individual may respond to genetically individualised treatments to universally recognised forms of morbidity, the healthy city needs to hold in its frame of vision at one time both global advances in medical science and local formations of urban life. This is as much a disposition as an epistemological position. It runs alongside a trend, witnessed in several parts of the world, to consider what it means to figure the urban as an ethically charged laboratory. In cities structured by particular path dependencies and lock-ins, interventions in public health demand a reflexivity mirroring unique circumstances and universal principles simultaneously. Such an approach starts with the sense that research knowledges that are sensitive to complex systems logics might prompt reconfigurations of the urban commons through interventions that share a disposition of the experimental.

Experimentation and intervention in the twenty-first-century city
Globally we have seen a growing appeal to an experimental urbanism (Evans, Karvone and Raven, 2016). A proliferation of urban living laboratories and city observatories have with varying degrees of success and very different ethical, commercial and state combinations built on such approaches to link research knowledge with policy praxis (Keith and Headlam, 2017; Marvin and Silver, 2016). In principle such laboratories involve situated and engaged research in specific contexts. Their work builds on, influences and is in turn influenced by the particular articulations of urban form. They are not straightforwardly sites for randomised or systemic testing of specific procedures or infrastructures. Instead, following the logic of complex systems theory, the situational limits of scaling imply that these forms of experimentation may operate differently at different scales. As the eminent ecologist Fikrek Berkes argues, in multilevel complex systems it is not always possible simply to scale up or scale down interventions, precisely because the non-linearity of processes of emergence may generate very different consequences at different scales vertically, horizontally and across time scales (Berkes, 2017).

Living laboratories and observatories are structured differently according to interest group and geography. They range from private-sector-driven sites of market testing to third-sector drives for citizen empowerment through open data to partnership structures of city government and urban stakeholders. Geographies of different approaches reflect different national political cultures. So the Scandinavian stakeholder partnership laboratories of Helsinki and Copenhagen differ significantly from the state-driven natural experiments increasingly deployed in neoclassical economics-driven research, the randomised control tests of medical work or the attempts to harvest even the most basic data on cities dominated by multiple informalities in many of the cities of the global south. Many of the institutions in the European Network of Living Labs look significantly different from city laboratories in Johannesburg and Mexico City, which in turn are similar in some ways to but different in many other ways from ostensibly similar institutions in Shenzhen or Singapore (Keith and Calzada, 2018).

What laboratories and observatories do share is a commitment to the practical deployment of new knowledge to locally informed city conditions. They take as a starting point the problem, particularly pronounced in public health and identified in the introduction to this volume, that devices such as randomised control trials and conventional experimental frames are ethically challenged in the twenty-first-century city. Research findings and policy interventions that flatten geographical and historical context may form a foundational form of the universal but are valid only as far as the historically particular and the geographically different are causally insignificant or irrelevant. In contrast, urban laboratories generally promote city interventions that are consciously both reflexive and tentative and potentially bridge divisions that reflect more established forms of urban expertise.

This is because alternative forms of urban expertise, different ways of 'knowing' the city, may each be powerful in their own hermetic context but lack incommensurable core measures of value and worth to facilitate exchange between them. For example, in the cities of industrial modernity a series of 'urban professions' have developed over time, dividing the governance of the city into professionally credentialised and formally recognised skillsets. Functionally powerful and technocratically effective in structuring the nineteenth-century city, they also are the source of forms of expertise that at times make the metropolis visible through lenses generating landscapes and logics that appear at times hard to reconcile. As one of the first countries to have urbanised, the United Kingdom (UK) provides a case in point. Credentialised by the crown, the *Royal* Institute of Chartered Surveyors, the *Royal* (sic) Town Planning Institute and the *Royal* Institute of British Architects provide powerful sources of legitimation and institutional power for their professions. They also promote sometimes rival ways of seeing the city, plural rationalities for organising the metropolis. They are powerful in promoting institutional interests and professional standards, sometimes less so in promoting crossover understandings between architects and planners, engineers, surveyors and health professionals.

In contrast, in cities that are driving the major urbanisations of the twenty-first century the professional boundaries are at times more permeable, allowing opportunities for citizens to see the city differently or even transcend systemic lock-ins. In this sense an experimental disposition is at times as significant as the nationally specific institutional forms of laboratories and observatories, particularly in a domain such as public health.

In the city of Cali in Colombia, the academic epidemiologist Rodrigo Guerrero in the first of his two periods of mayoralty in 1992 famously created an urban laboratory specifically to consider urban violence as an epidemic, synthesising social sciences and medical science when combining cartographies of pattern with social sciences of neighbourhood to shape policy interventions. And in Medellin under the mayoral regime of Sergio Fajardo from 2012 to 2016, the city developed a practice of *social urbanism*, led by the architect and planner Alejandro Echeverri, founder of the Colombian research group URBAM, which was akin in many ways to a related form of 'urban acupuncture'. In measuring different regimes of *valuing* economic growth, rational planning or automobile mobilities, social urbanism prioritised an attempt to diminish the profoundly unequal configurations of city life that characterised the history of the city. As in many parts of the globe, the city demonstrated a stark separation of the majority populations of informal barrios from the formal city subject to cadastration, real estate markets, established infrastructure, automobile logics and enforced property rights. The addressing of the pressing demand to transcend the spatial segregation of rich from poor in informal settlements led to the imperative to subvert conventional transport studies logics of mass transit provision through the landmark construction of a cable-car system that began to bridge the separation of the formal city and the sequestered and informal barrios. Recognition of the social capital and cultural dimensions of mobility addresses specifically the social equity dimensions of integrating the city, building welfare, social and cultural facilities along the route of the cable car and reconfiguring the staging of gender relations and the calculus of safety in the city (Kaufmann, Bergman and Joye, 2004; Levy, 2013; Levy et al., 2017). Along the intersections of the cable-car network, the city focused public health, education and community engagement. Subverting an 'either/or' choice of either optimal transport mobility or rationally distributed public health real estate, Medellin's social urbanism appropriated an innovative form of city mobility to build bridges across divided social worlds. Originally proposed as a driver of city tourism, counter-intuitively in some senses the Medellin cable cars are now regarded as an instrument of social inclusion and are recognised as one of the more successful infrastructural interventions in cities of the global south.

They are seen as working well because the metrics of their 'success' – how value is calculated – are measured by the imaginative leap in their design and the creative outcomes that they generated. Cable cars displaced the spatial fix, or geographical lock-in, of separation caused by social segregation through technological intervention. They revolve around a recognition that policy intervention needs to recognise what might appear to be 'clumsy' or sub-optimal but works with the rhythms and speed of the city itself. Medellin also highlights the different measures of *value* and *worth* that are at stake in such intervention, a phenomenon that is also identified in an intermediate technological intervention in the landscape of Kathmandu. In arguing for the importance for an imaginary of future urbanism that is geographically sensitive, Thompson and Beck (2014) make these arguments explicitly in their discussion of the plural rationalities at stake in the construction of the Kathmandu Battendra milkway when assessing the values that define an effective deployment of technological disruption. Complicating the conventional distinction between hierarchies and markets, they taxonomise a distinction between the logics of four ideal typical voices addressing emergent urbanisms, four future dispositions. The hierarchist voice of control and planning contrasts with the individualist voice of the utility-optimising individual, an egalitarian voice that they suggest places distributive goals above all others and a fatalist voice that treats the future as a hand of cards that is dealt and beyond control.

Thompson and Beck highlight how before the milkway was built villagers on the periphery of the city boiled milk down to *khuwa*, a longer-lasting but less valuable condensed form. Kathmandu has grown faster than Industrial Revolution Manchester, with a population of almost three million imminent in the broadly conceived metropolitan area, challenging the transport of *khuwa*. But the new milkway reduced a five-hour journey to twenty minutes, generating an income rise of 30 per cent. It also reduced the negative externalities of the *khuwa* production, the ecological damage of the wood-cutting to boil the *khuwa*, the opening-up of a market gardening cluster and the development of social inclusion in economic growth. And yet the milkway was what Thompson and Beck describe as a 'clumsy' solution to a 'wicked' problem. In analytical terms they suggest it lacked elegance. Thompson and Beck (2014: 22) quote the anthropologist Madhukar Upadhya as suggesting that 'The ropeway has thus become not only a transport system but a community-wide benefit provider, thanks to the social capital it has itself generated.' And yet the milkway was constructed in the face of opposition from technocratically inclined European Union donors and authoritarian government alike, who had prioritised what they saw as a technologically defined crisis of land management and a conventionally described model of economic development.

The path-dependent starting point of the Kathmandu example opens up the city as a site of potential, an arena of possibility. It does not contradict the economically optimal, but it drives change through the use of different lenses to define the *problem* to which policy intervention is addressed. A problem of economic sustainability is redefined through a lens of public health that also addresses challenges of ecological disruption and deforestation. It is not a coincidence that both the opportunities and some of the most interesting examples of how a careful understanding of the dynamics of urban systems help to generate a cautious overcoming of path dependence emerge from the cities of what we might conventionally understand as the global south. These forms of creativity and invention litter the writing of scholars such as AbdouMaliq Simone in cities as diverse as Dhaka and Phnom Penh (Simone and Pieterse, 2017; Simone, 2019) and are at the heart of an urbanism that Ravi Sundaram (2010) has described as a form of 'pirate modernity' or Gautam Bhan (2019) has suggested is a distinctive form of 'southern urbanism'.

Pragmatic commensuration? Law, property rights, 'mohalla' clinics and healthy squatting in Delhi

Bhan's work has foregrounded not only how the practices of the informal city demonstrate similarities across the global south but also that health policy interventions demand a pragmatic understanding of location. In the example we first raised in the introduction to this volume, he considers the rapid proliferation of city health centres in contemporary Delhi. Bhan argues that 'the squat' in India can be understood only situationally, as a paradigmatic Indian southern practice. As a form of city practice squatting in India represents an urban intervention that invokes a notion of legitimacy as much as one of legality, following Partha Chatterjee's (2004) landmark framing of a 'politics of the governed' that appeals to the values of legal discourse rooted in the appeal to constitutional rights to challenge the legitimacy of urban exclusionary processes. In the Indian city such practice sustains poor people's movements that create 'rights-bearing citizens in the sense imagined by the constitution' (Chatterjee, 2004: 38) in juxtaposition to realities confronted by excluded settlements on the margins of society with tenuous hold on a right to the city, the right to have somewhere to live.

Bhan describes how in the complex political cartography of early twenty-first-century Delhi local political control by progressive forces uses the practice of squatting to establish a plurality of new 'mohalla' health centres, frequently occupying sidewalk locations arbitrarily and with tendentious claims to legal tenure. Evocatively he writes:

> Consider this set of practices: building a 'temporary' structure; using a particular set of materials and construction techniques that reflect an uncertain temporality; building knowingly in tension with regimes of law, property and planning (the health minister did not deny that one could not build on a sidewalk); proceeding without resolving these tensions or knowing if a resolution is possible; and simultaneously defending one's occupation on moral and ethical grounds (this is, after all, a public clinic) as well as technicalities (this is a 'temporary' structure). This is a familiar set of claims and processes. The government of Delhi is, to put it bluntly, squatting on the land of the North Delhi Municipal Corporation. It is entirely possible, reading the health minister's response, to argue that they know precisely that they are squatting. In responding as they did, one can argue that the AAP government is challenging the central government to demolish – in public space and public view – what is, after all, not a form of private appropriation, but by a public health centre. Legally, the municipal corporation is right. Yet the clinic draws its staying power more through a claim to legitimacy than to legality. (Bhan, 2019: 7)

While couched in the language of 'southern urbanism', Bhan's analysis also points to something more simple: that interventions in urban form are always shaped by geographical and historical context; they generate mutations of the urban system that might share similar logics and conjure very different outcomes. In this context effective policy design has no choice but to work with the grain of historically and geographically specific property rights and constitutional claims, recognising the moments of the universal alongside the power of specific in shaping the emergent. As Bhan goes on to suggest:

> [my] intention here is not to debate which government is 'right', nor to draw a simplistic equivalence between a mohalla clinic and a pavement dweller. It is to show that squatting as a practice has a set of logics that make it both effective and necessary for reaching certain outcomes in the specific historical and spatial contexts of Southern urbanisation. Taking Southern practice seriously means seeing squatting not just in its tensions with formal logics of law and planning, nor merely in the material forms of housing, but as mode of practice that embraces uncertainty, measures itself against limited temporalities, and operates to move forward incrementally in any way it can. This mode of practice is claimed here as an equal possibility for state action – for policies, programmes and plans – and not just for subaltern urban residents. To use Solomon Benjamin's conceptualisation, squatting is a practice that can allow even planners within state structures to become occupancy urbanists. This results in new forms of planning practice from within the state apparatus. (Bhan, 2019: 7)

Bhan's argument powerfully foregrounds both a critical disposition and also a sense of the propositonal. The combinations of global problems shaped by local context that prefigure a politics of geographical scale also complement a logic of urban experimentation. This demands in turn an imperative of humility: cities that aspire to be truly 'smart' are those that recognise their own histories and understand their presents, shaping bespoke interventions that synthesise new urban science and local knowledges while acknowledging transparently what fails as well as what might succeed.

While not driven by institutional forms of city laboratories or observatories, the public health drivers of change in Kathmandu, Medellin and Delhi share a particularly experimental sensibility, one that is seen on an even grander scale in the opening-up of the cities of China in the post-1978 period. What has been described as 'local state capitalism' in China has also driven the cautious attempt to 'cross the river one stone at a time', as Deng Xiaoping carefully described the opening-up process in China from 1978 (Keith et al., 2014). In a nation like China with territorial scale and population numbers much greater than those of the whole of Europe and Northern America combined, Confucian tensions between the governance centre and dispersed geographies repeat through the centuries. In China's devolved system, while the party does not surrender power, the cities become real-time experiments as different ways of shaping urban futures are trialled. Some have already argued that the rhetorical commitment to design an urbanism of the paradoxical socialist marketplace that Deng espoused should be taken more seriously than Western commentators and most urbanists have suggested. Deng's model grew from the evolution of Special Economic Zones, which trialled different forms of urban economic growth models, from the accelerated urban growth of 'Shenzhen speed' (Shenzhen sudu 深圳速度) of the Pearl River Delta, which grew a city of 280,000 in small villages to a metropolis of ten to fifteen million in thirty years, to the Chongqing Model of egalitarian growth attempted by the disgraced 'princeling' Bo Xilai, whose model of change was however celebrated by left scholars in China (Arrighi, 2007; Cui, 2011; Frenkiel, 2010) and beyond.

More significantly, the record of China's urbanism over now more than four decades represents both the continuity of long traditions of uncertain relations between the centre of a 1.4 billion 'civilisation state' in Beijing and varying degrees of local autonomy. The experimental disposition of bespoke urban policy interventions at the micro-scale of acupuncture and social urbanism are seen in China at the macro-scale of whole city systems that are allowed a sense of earned autonomy to trial different policy solutions to generic urban problems. These 'experiments' with models of urban change that have emerged from the post-1978 processes in China may or may not survive the attempts by Xi Jinping to recentralise many of the instruments of policy control, but represent some of the more significant and less explored ways in which the city as a whole becomes a laboratory for 'solution-oriented urbanism'.

We consequently argue that considering the global urbanisms of public health imperatives demands a way of thinking that integrates the domains of new urban sciences and historically and geographically contextual knowledges. The power of prediction (P), the non-linear logic of emergence (E) and the commensuration of new forms of adopted knowledge (A) generated by disruptive innovation structured the introduction to this volume. In the conclusion we have focused on the imperative to develop new forms of knowledge exchange (K) between citizens, cities and science that are at the heart of what might be a new urban imaginary. This imaginary we have described elsewhere as a PEAK Urban approach to the sorts of challenges presented by the public health dilemmas addressed in the substantive chapters of this volume.[1] In essence such an imaginary might rest on a sense of the power of an interdisciplinary space that bridges natural sciences, social sciences and humanities, while also sustaining a sense of humility in respecting diverse local histories, contextual geographies and path-dependent futures that define the diversity of twenty-first-century urban life.

The chapters of this volume in very different ways share many of these approaches, understanding the importance of urban context in shaping transport interventions (Schwanen and Nixon in Chapter 4) or food systems (Smit in Chapter 6), health services in the 'broken city' (Ortega and Wenceslau in Chapter 7), the cultural traffic between cities of the north and south (Mcilwaine et al. in Chapter 3), and the logic of systems thinking in qualifying the capacity of straightforwardly technocratic approaches to water and sewage network development (Iossifova in Chapter 5). In very different ways the return to a form of vitalism in Nikolas Rose's framing of urban mental health (Chapter 2) and the historical context of racialised injustice and the roots of structural violence in urban Brazil today (Soares in Chapter 8) share a sense of both path dependency and propensity in shaping the pathologies of public health. They also share a commitment to a framing of social scientific research that continues to foreground the critical dispositions that emerge from the ethical crucible of urban life alongside a facility to engage with the natural sciences in general and the logics of medicine in particular. Whether through new institutional forms such as urban laboratories or city observatories, the continental scale of governance variation between cities in twenty-first-century China or the diverse creativities of 'social urbanism', 'acupunctural urbanism' or 'southern urban practice', such approaches also demand that an experimental sense of city propensity demands a reconfigured relationship between 'blue skies' research, the ivory tower and the social context of the cities that drive human dwelling for the twenty-first century.

Note

1 See the collaborative programme PEAK Urban linking studies of urban futures across China, Colombia, India and South Africa (www.peak-urban. org).

References

Arrighi, G. (2007). *Adam Smith in Beijing: Lineages of the twenty-first century*. London and New York: Verso.

Berkes, F. (2017). Environmental governance for the Anthropocene? Social-ecological systems, resilience, and collaborative learning. *Sustainability*, 9(7), art. 1232.

Bhan, G. (2019). Notes on a southern urban practice. *Environment and Urbanization*, 31(2): 1–19.

Chatterjee, P. (2004). *The politics of the governed: Reflections on popular politics in most of the world*. New York: Columbia University Press.

Cui, Z. (2011). Partial intimations of the coming whole: The Chongqing experiment in light of the theories of Henry George, James Meade, and Antonio Gramsci. *Modern China*, 37(6): 1–16.

Evans, J., Karvone, A., and Raven, R. (2016). *The experimental city: New modes and prospects of urban transformation*. London: Routledge.

Frenkiel, E. (2010). *From scholar to official: Cui Zhiyuan and Chongqing City's local experimental policy*. Ideas&books.net, https://booksandideas.net/IMG/pdf/20101206_Cui_Zhiyuan_EN.pdf (last accessed 1 November 2019).

Kaufmann, V., Bergman, M., and Joye, D. (2004). Motility: Mobility as capital. *International Journal of Urban and Regional Research*, 28(4): 745–56.

Keith, M., and Calzada, I. (2018). *Back to the 'urban commons'? Amidst social innovation through new cooperative forms in Europe*. Oxford: Urban Transformations.

Keith, M., and Headlam, N. (2017). *Comparative international urban and living labs: The Urban Living Global Challenge*. Report for Oxford City Futures: Spring Symposium.

Keith, M., Lash, S., Arnoldi, J., and Rooker, T. (2014). *China constructing capitalism: Economic life and urban change*. London and New York: Routledge.

Levy, C. (2013). Transport, diversity, and the socially just city: The significance of gender relations. In J. Dávila (ed.), *Urban mobility and poverty: Lesson from Medellin and Socaha, Colombia*, 23–30. London: Development Planning Unit, UCL.

Levy, B.S., Sidel, V.W., and Patz, J.A. (2017). Climate change and collective violence. *Annual Review of Public Health*, 38(1): 241–57.

Marvin, S., and Silver, J. (2016). The urban laboratory and emerging sites of urban experimentation. In J.K. Evans, A. Karvonen, A., and Raven, R. (eds), *The experimental city*, 47–60. London and New York: Routledge.

Simone, A. (2019). *Improvised lives: Rhythms of endurance in an urban south (after the postcolonial)*. London: Polity Press.

Simone. A., and Pieterse, E. (2017). *New urban worlds: Inhabiting dissonant times*. Medford: Polity Press.

Sundaram, R. (2010). Pirate modernity: Delhi's media urbanism. Abingdon and New York: Routledge.

Thompson, M., and Beck, M.B. (2014). *Coping with change: Urban resilience, sustainability, adaptability and path dependence.* Future of Cities working paper. London: Foresight, Government Office for Science.

Index

access
   mobility and 84, 86
   walking and cycling 90–1, 94
accessibility 84–5, 91
actor-network theory (ANT) 109–10
actuarial risk 18–19
ageing populations 108
agency of infrastructure 12, 16–17, 24
agriculture 133, 134, 135, 137
alcohol outlets 131–2
Allen, Pete 9–10
allostatic load 43–5
Amerindian perspectivism 182, 185–6
Andrew, Caroline 56, 71
antidepressant medication 155, 158
appropriation 84–5, 86, 94–6
apps 38–9
Arendt, Hannah 20
Aristotle 12, 81
'asphalt'/'hill'
   as moral economies 161–3
   in Rio de Janeiro 149–54
   therapeutic approaches in 154–60
   use of categories 149–50, 163–4
assemblages 12, 83, 85, 86, 93–4, 97
automobility 88–9

Bai, Xuemei 110–11
Beck, M. Bruce 204–5
'behavioural sinks' 42
Bergman, Manfred Max 84–5
Bhan, Gautam 23–4, 205–7
bicycle maintenance/repair 92–3
big data 6, 8–9, 198
biological and sociocultural approaches 11, 35–6, 37–8
biological localities 48–9
biopolitics 36, 39–40, 46–8, 49

bodily experiences
   of depression 153, 161
   social sciences and 111–12
Boiteux, Luciana 180
Botswana food security 135
Brazil
   institutions 178–80
   mental health in 147, 148, 149
   migration within 189–91
   violence 175
   see also Rio de Janeiro; São Paulo, Brazil
'buffering' of stress 45–6
building/dwelling perspectives 191

cable cars 203–4
Calhoun, John 42
Canguilhem, Georges 11
Cannon, Walter 42
capabilities
   access and 91
   functionings and 82–3, 86, 94, 97–8
   time-spaces 27, 80, 83–5, 91–3, 98
   urban space and 89–90
   walking as 95–6
   wellbeing 80, 85–6
Capabilities Approaches (CA) 80, 82–3, 85–6
Cape Town, South Africa 130–1, 132, 136
CAPS (Center for Psychosocial Care) 157–8
causality
   propensity and 24
   urban mental health 40–1
   in urban scholarship 6–8, 9–12
Centre for Psychosocial Care (CAPS) 157–8
Chatterjee, Partha 206
childhood, toxic stress in 44, 46

Index

China
  health provision trade-offs 21–3
  urban change and sanitation 104–9, 112, 113–14
  urbanism 207–8
Chisikone Market, Kitwe 138
cities
  defining 4
  diversity of 3
  metabolism of 2–3, 4–5
  seeing like a city 14
citizen-led initiatives 80, 87–8, 98
city commons 1–2, 198
Clark, David A. 82–3
closed-loop sanitation systems 105–6, 107, 113–14
cognitive appropriation 85
  see also appropriation
commensuration 6, 17–24, 205–9
common pool resources 2, 5–6
commons
  city 1–2, 198
  tragedy of the 2
competencies
  mobility and 85, 86
  walking and cycling 91–4, 95–6
complexity theory 111, 115
complex systems 2–4, 5–13, 198–9, 201
Consuming Urban Poverty research project 124
credit in informal shops 131
crime, fear of 94–5
criminal justice 178–80
cycling
  citizen-led initiatives 80–1, 87–8
  cultivating potential for 88–96
  São Paulo and London 86–8

Dar es Salaam, Tanzania 21
data analytics 8–9
data-rich urban science 198
defibrillators 13, 14–15
Delhi, India 24, 205–7
Deng Xiaoping 21, 200, 207–8
density 42–3
depression
  case studies 156–60
  symptoms and determinants 151–4
  therapeutic approaches 154–6
  urban living 147–9
de Souza Santos, Andreza Aruska, chapters by 1–34, 198–210
determinism 9, 11–12, 37
dietary diversity 124, 134
disabilities, people with 90–1
disadvantaged individuals/groups
  citizen-led initiatives 87–8, 96
  further research 97–8

wellbeing 79–80, 90–1, 92, 94
domestic violence 63–6, 69–70
  see also violence against women and girls (VAWG)
drinking water 135–6, 138
drug dealing 177–8, 180
drug use 71, 177–8
dwelling/building perspectives 191–2

Echeverri, Alejandro 203
ecological model of gender-based violence (GBV) 58
emergence 6, 11, 13–17, 20–1, 23–4
entwined becoming 97
epigenetics 37, 38, 44
ethical dilemmas 18–21, 23–4
ethnographic approaches 150–1, 163–4
eudaimonic conceptions of wellbeing 81–2, 85, 89, 95, 97
Evans, Yara
  chapter by 55–78
  discussion 25–6, 199, 209
experimental thinking 6
experimentation 10, 201–5, 207–8
expertise
  clustering of 15–16
  commensuration of 6, 17, 202

Fajardo, Sergio 203
Family Health Strategy (FHS) 150–2
Fassin, Didier 36, 162–3
fear
  of crime 94–5
  women's right to the city 66–7, 72–3
Ferguson, James 20–1
Flamm, Michael 84
flushing toilets 104, 107
food deserts 134, 140
Food Environment Classification Tool 125
food environments
  in African cities 126–9, 139–40
  broader urban environment 132–3
  concept of 124–6
  health and 125, 133–6
  marketplaces 129–32
food policy councils 138–9
food safety 132, 135–6, 138
food security/insecurity 123–4, 128, 133, 134–9
food swamps 134, 140
'foodways' 126, 139
forced labour 68
formality/informality 126–7
Freirean theory 188
fuel sources 135–6
functionings 82–3, 86, 94, 96–8
'fundamental causes' 41, 45

Galea, Sandro 44–5
gangs
  justice and 179
  prisons and 178
  violence 67, 70, 172
Garcia, Afrânio 189
gender-based violence (GBV)
  causes of 68–71
  conceptualising 56–60
  health, gender and the right to the city 71–4
  multidimensionality 63–5
  research methodologies 60–2
  spaces of 65–8
  tolerance of 59, 73–4
  urban living and 55–6
general adaptation syndrome 42
geomapping 38–9
Gilroy, Paul 174
Glass, Thomas A. 10
Global Mental Health 148–9, 153, 164
Goldberg, David 161
Goldstein, Kurt 11
governance
  of cities 1–3
  historic public health 4–5
  urban food environments 138–9
Guerrero, Rodrigo 203

Hägerstrand, Torsten 84
Hansen, Pelle G. 19–20
Hardin, Garrett 2
Harré, Rom 12
health care
  distribution of infrastructure 13, 14, 16
  informal care and 47
  inverse care law 163
  Rio de Janeiro 150–2
  trade-offs in China 21–3
health centres 206
Healthy China 2030 106
hedonic conceptions of wellbeing 81, 82–3, 85, 93, 95, 97
Hegel, Friedrich 173–4
Heise, Lori 58
'hill'/'asphalt'
  as moral economies 161–3
  in Rio de Janeiro 149–54
  therapeutic approaches in 154–60
  use of categories 149–50, 163–4
hospital distribution 16
housing 7–8, 57, 191
hukou system 21–2
human practice 111
human trafficking 68

identity and migration 189–90, 192
imaginary 200–1, 208–9

immigration status 69
incarceration 177–8, 179–80
India
  sanitation 23–4
  squatting in Delhi 205–7
individuality 187, 193–5
inequalities
  Brazil 148, 187
  mental health and 46
  networked cities 103
  reproduction of 176, 178–80, 187–9, 193
  Rio de Janeiro 149–54, 175
  wellbeing and 79–80, 90
informality 126–7
informal settlements 129, 132–3, 136, 137–8
informal shops 127, 131–2, 137
infrastructure
  agency of 24
  materiality of 15–16
  in networked city 103
  propensity of 13–17
  sanitation 102, 105–8, 109, 114
  in traditional marketplaces 130
  urban food environments and 137–8
Ingold, Tim 191
institutional racism 178–80, 181
institutional violence 67–8, 69–70
insurance 18–19, 22–3
Internet of Things 107
intersectionality 58–9, 69
intimate partner violence (IPV) 65–6, 71
inverse care law 163
Iossifova, Deljana
  chapter by 102–22
  discussion 27, 200
'I–You' social dynamics 184–5, 193

Jacobs, Jane 94
James, C.L.R. 174
Joelsson, Irmelin 21
Joye, Dominique 84–5
Jubilee Market, Kisumu 129–30
justice, access to 193

ka tables 127
  see also informal shops
Kathmandu, Nepal 204–5
Kaufmann, Vincent 84–5, 97
Keith, Michael, chapters by 1–34, 198–210
Khayelitsha, South Africa 130–1
Kibuye Market, Kisumu 129
Kisumu, Kenya
  food environments 127–9
  food safety 136
  governance 138
  marketplaces 129–30

Index

Kitwe, Zambia 137, 138
Krenzinger, Miriam
  chapter by 55–78
  discussion 25–6, 199, 209
landscape 191
land-use zoning 131, 132, 136–9
Lefebvre, Henri 20
LGBTQ+ people, violence against 67
life sciences 36–7, 46
Link, Bruce 41, 44–5
living laboratories/observatories 201–3, 207–8
local food 133
local government
  role in traditional marketplaces 130
  urban food environment 138–9
local state capitalism 207–8
Lock, Margaret 48–9
lock-ins 12, 16, 23–4, 201, 204
London
  Bangladeshi family housing 7–8
  causes of VAWG 68–71
  cycling and walking 86–94, 95–6
  multidimensionality of VAWG 63–5
  research methodologies 60–1
  spaces of VAWG 65–8
  urban VAWG and the right to the city 71–4

magnetic resonance imaging (MRI) scanners 15–16
malnutrition 124, 134
Manning, Nick 44
Maré, Rio de Janeiro
  causes of VAWG 68–71
  multidimensionality of VAWG 63–5
  research methodologies 61–2
  spaces of VAWG 65–8
  urban VAWG and the right to the city 71–4
markets/marketplaces
  informal shops 131–2
  street food vendors 132
  supermarkets 130–1
  traditional 127, 128, 129–30
Marmot, Michael 38
master-slave relationship 182–4
materiality of infrastructure 15–16
McEwen, Bruce 43–4
McEwen, Craig 44
McIlwaine, Cathy
  chapter by 55–78
  discussion 25–6, 199, 209
mechanisms
  beyond social factors 38
  importance of 41
  stress as 38, 42

Medellin, Colombia 203–4
mental health
  the city and 35–6
  government programmes 39–40, 47
  informal care 47
  mechanisms 41–5
  migrant women 72
  social determinants 38
  transformations in care 150–4
  urban living and 147–8
migrant women 60–1, 63–5, 67–70, 72
migration
  access to toilets 114
  within Brazil 189–91, 192
  mental health and 35
  violence against women and girls (VAWG) 58–9
violence as driver of 68
military police 179–81
milkway 204–5
miscegenation 188
mobility
  access to health resources 15
  capabilities and 96, 97–8
  concept of 84–5
  wellbeing-mobility nexus 85–6
  wellbeing and 80–1, 88–90
modelling 9–10
mohalla clinics 206–7
moral anthropology 162–3
moral dilemmas 18–21, 23–4
moral economies 156–60, 161–3
Mors, Susan Buck 174
motility 80, 84–5, 86, 94, 97–8
Mozambique 135
murder 175–7

Nairobi, Kenya 124
National Urban and Rural Environmental Sanitation Clean Action Plan (2015–2020) 106
networked cities 102–4
neuroscience 36–7
New Type Urbanisation Plan (2014–20) 108
New York 39–40, 47
night soil collection 105–6
Nixon, Denver V.
  chapter by 79–101
  discussion 26–7, 198–200, 209
non-intimate partner violence (non-IPV) 57
nudging and individual rights 18, 19–20
nutrition environments 125

obesity 124, 133–4
obesogenic environment thesis 134

obligations 3, 19, 20, 198
ontological dualities 181–7, 188–9, 192, 193, 195
Ortega, Francisco
  chapter by 147–70
  discussion 28–9, 199, 209
Ostrom, Elinor 2
Other, the 181, 184, 185–6, 193–5
overcrowding 42–3, 57

Palmeira, Moacir 189
path dependencies 12, 13–14, 24, 182–3, 201, 205
Patriotic Health Campaign 105–6
PEAK Urban approach 208
'Pedro' (case study) 158–60
person-centred consultations 155, 157, 163, 164
Phelan, Jo 41, 45
pit latrines 104, 108
planning
  differing measures of value 202–3, 204, 205–7
  mobility and access 84
  sanitation 102–3, 110, 113–14
  stress research and 42–3
  urban food environments 126–7, 129, 137, 139–40
policing 176–7, 178–81
policy *see* urban policy
politics of the governed 206
pollution 37, 81, 84, 107, 114
potential outcomes frameworks 10
poverty
  causality and 7–8, 40–1
  criminalisation of 178–80, 195
  mental health and 38, 46, 148, 153
  violence against women and girls (VAWG) 58
power relations 68–9
practice theory 111–13, 115
prediction 6, 9–13
prevention 4, 47, 198
primary health care
  distribution of infrastructure 13, 14, 16
  informal care and 47
  inverse care law 163
  Rio de Janeiro 150–2
private/public spheres 56, 57
professions 202–3
propensity 11, 12, 13–17, 24
provincialising urban scholarship 110–11, 114–15
public goods 17, 20
public health
  defining 4
  framing the city through 198–9, 205

public interest 2, 198
public spaces 66, 70, 88–90, 94–5
racism
  class and 181, 187–8
  institutional/structural 178–80, 193
  Rio de Janeiro 172–4
  violence against women and girls (VAWG) 64
Rapoport, Amos 43
'Raquel' (case study) 156–8
Rawls publicity principle 19–20
real estate of health care 16
reflexivity 201, 202
refrigeration 132
regime change 192–3
research *see* urban scholarship
research methodologies
  citizen-led cycling and walking initiatives 87–8
  mental health 38–9, 151–2
  violence against women and girls (VAWG) 60–2
resilience 153, 155, 163
Retail Food Environment Index 125
rights
  health provision trade-offs 21–3
  individual 17–21
right to the city
  excluded settlements 206
  gender and 56, 59, 65, 71–4
  limits to 20
  in policy design 17
  Rio de Janeiro
    causes of violence against women and girls (VAWG) 68–71
    'hill' and 'asphalt' in 149–54
    mental health case studies 156–60
    multidimensionality of VAWG 63–5
    murder victims 176
    research methodologies 61–2
    spaces of VAWG 65–8
    state violence 180–1
    therapeutic approaches to mental health 154–6
    urban VAWG and the right to the city 71–4
    violence 175
Robeyns, Ingrid 97
Rose, Nikolas
  chapter by 35–54
  discussion 11, 25, 199, 209
rural life and identity 189–90

Sandel, Michael 19
sanitation
  food safety 135–6, 138
  impact of poor 23–4

Index

networked cities 103–4
towards a practice approach 109–15
urban change in China 104–9
violence against women and girls (VAWG) 57
São Paulo, Brazil
 cycling and walking 86–92, 94–6
 Megacity Mental Health Survey 148, 149
 mental health 148
Schwanen, Tim
 chapter by 79–101
 discussion 26–7, 198–200, 209
Science and Technology Studies (STS) 11
self-monitoring 18–20
Selye, Hans 42
Sen, Amartya 80, 82–3
service-networked sanitation 105–6, 107, 113–14
sewage-based sanitation 105, 108, 114
sexual abuse 71
sexual harassment 66, 68, 70
Shove, Elizabeth 112–13
Simone, Maliq 205
skills 91–4
 see also competencies
Skov, Katrine L. 19–20
Skov, Laurits R. 19–20
slavery
 dual ontologies 183–7, 193
 ongoing significance 187–8
 path dependencies of 182–3
Smit, Warren
 chapter by 123–46
 discussion 27–8, 200, 209
Soares, Luiz Eduardo
 biography and research 171–5
 chapter by 171–97
 discussion 12, 26, 29, 199, 209
social capital 45–7, 203
social determinants
 of mental health 38, 41, 44–8, 151–4, 164
 of violence against women and girls (VAWG) 57–8
social integration
 bicycle repair 93–4
 time-spaces 83
social networks
 depression and 152–3, 154, 163
 migration and 189–90
social sciences
 biological roots of 37–8
 bodily experiences and 111–12
 stress research 46
social urbanism 203–4
sociocultural and biological approaches 11, 35–6, 37–8

socio-eco-technical approaches 111
sociotechnical approaches 109–10
solid waste 136
'somatisation' 153
Sousa Silva, Eliana
 chapter by 55–78
 discussion 25–6, 199, 209
South Africa 20–1, 130–1, 135
southern urbanism 23–4, 205–6
space, wellbeing and mobility 88–90
spaza shops 127
 see also informal shops
Special Economic Zones 208
speed
 of access to health resources 13, 14–16
 of urban change 12–13
squatting 205–7
squat toilets 104
state violence 180–1
Stellar, Elliot 43–4
street food vendors 128, 132, 135, 138
street lighting 57
stress 41–8
structural violence 56, 57–9, 65, 69–71, 74
Sundaram, Ravi 205
supermarkets 130–1, 135
supernatural, the 185–6
Sustainable Development Goals 59, 107
systems
 complex 2–4, 5–13, 198–9, 201
 health care 17–24
 metropolitan/urban 6, 7, 24
 of systems 3–4, 9, 198
systems approach 111, 115

technological change
 health systems and 13–17
 individual rights and 18–21
temporality 191–2
temporary structures 206–7
therapeutic time-spaces 84
Thompson, Michael 204–5
ThriveNYC 39–40, 47
time-spaces 83–4, 85–6, 93
Titmuss, Richard 20
Toilet Revolution 106–7, 114
toilets 104, 106–7, 108
 see also sanitation
tourism 106–7
tradition and territory 192
transnationality 55, 68, 69, 74
transport networks 70, 132–3
'tuck shops' *see* informal shops
Tudor Hart, Julian 163

UN-Habitat New Urban Agenda (NUA) 59
UN-Habitat Safer Cities 59

United Kingdom health care distribution 14–15, 16
'unit groups' 154, 160, 162
urban agriculture 133, 134, 135, 137
'Urban Brain' research programme 36, 48
urban commons 1–2
urban food environments
  in African cities 126–9, 139–40
  broader urban environment 132–3
  concept of 124–6
  health and 133–6
  marketplaces 129–32
urban imaginaries 200–1, 208–9
urbanisation
  Brazil 189–91
  China 104–9, 114
  gender and 56–7, 59
urbanism
  global 12, 111, 208–9
  social 203–4
  Southern 23–4, 206
urban justice 56
urban living laboratories 201–3, 207–8
urban policy
  context and design 205–7
  criminal justice 178–80
  evidence and experimentation 8, 10–11, 202–3, 204, 208
  mental health 39–40, 47
  networked cities 102–3
  sanitation 105–9, 113
urban scholarship
  causality in 6–8, 9–12
  data analysis in 8–9
  new configuration of 5–6, 24
  provincialising of 110–11, 114–15
urban violence 58, 66, 70–1, 203
user perspectives 39

value 6, 19–20, 22, 203–4
violence
  fear of 94–5
  incarceration for 177–8
  by the state 180–1
  urban 26, 58, 66, 70–1, 203
violence against women and girls (VAWG)
  causes of 68–71
  conceptualising 56–60
  health, gender and the right to the city 71–4

multidimensionality 63–5
research methodologies 60–2
spaces of 65–8
tolerance of 59, 73–4
urban living and 55–6
vitalism 11–12
Viveiros de Castro, Eduardo 182–3, 185–6, 187
Viswanath, Kalpana 56, 71

Waiselfisz, Julio Jacobo 175
walking
  citizen-led initiatives 80–1, 87–8
  cultivating potential for 88–96
  São Paulo and London 86–8
water-borne sanitation 103–4, 107–8, 114
wearable devices 18–20
welfare 20–1, 22
wellbeing
  concept of 79–80, 81–4
  mobility and space 88–90
  sustainable 110
  wellbeing-mobility nexus 85–6
  of women 56–7, 71–2, 74
Wenceslau, Leandro David
  chapter by 147–70
  discussion 28–9, 199, 209
wheelchair users 90–1
Whitzman, Carolyn 56, 71
wicked problems 23–4, 205
women
  causes of violence against women and girls (VAWG) 68–71
  conceptualising VAWG 56–60
  health and the right to the city 71–4
  multidimensionality of VAWG 63–5
  spaces of VAWG 65–8
  urban living and 55–6
  wellbeing of 56–7, 71–2, 74
workplace violence 66, 70, 72
World Health Organization (WHO) 5, 38
worth 6, 202–4
  see also value

Xi Jinping 22–3, 208

Zambia 127, 131, 133, 137–8

EU authorised representative for GPSR:
Easy Access System Europe, Mustamäe tee 50,
10621 Tallinn, Estonia
gpsr.requests@easproject.com

www.ingramcontent.com/pod-product-compliance
Ingram Content Group UK Ltd.
Pitfield, Milton Keynes, MK11 3LW, UK
UKHW011931180825
461986UK00006B/121